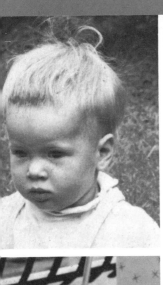
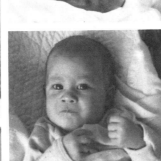
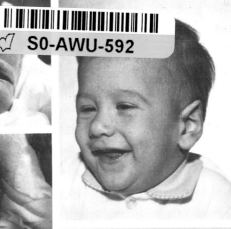
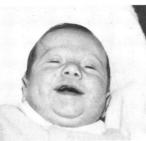

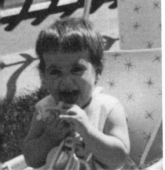
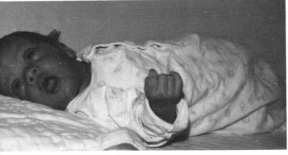
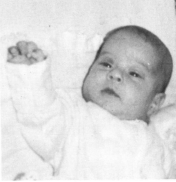
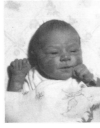
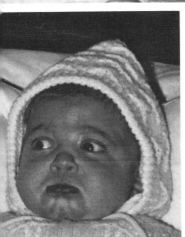
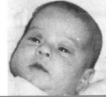
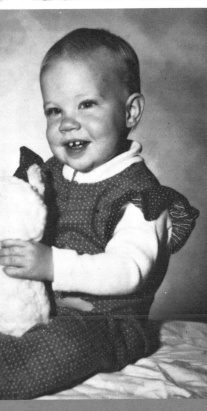

MALE
INFERTILITY

RICHARD D. AMELAR, M.D.

Professor of Clinical Urology
New York University School of Medicine
Attending Urologist
New York University Medical Center

LAWRENCE DUBIN, M.D.

Professor of Clinical Urology
New York University School of Medicine
Attending Urologist
New York University Medical Center

PATRICK C. WALSH, M.D.

Professor and Director
Department of Urology
The Johns Hopkins University School of Medicine;
Urologist-in-Chief
James Buchanan Brady Urological Institute
The Johns Hopkins Hospital

1977

W. B. SAUNDERS COMPANY • Philadelphia • London • Toronto

W. B. Saunders Company: West Washington Square
Philadelphia, Pa. 19105

1 St. Anne's Road
Eastbourne, East Sussex BN21 3UN, England

1 Goldthorne Avenue
Toronto, Ontario M8Z 5T9, Canada

Library of Congress Cataloging in Publication Data

Amelar, Richard D

Male infertility.

Includes index.

1. Sterility, Male.   I. Dubin, Lawrence, joint author.
II. Walsh, Patrick C., joint author.   III. Title.
[DNLM: 1. Sterility, Male. WJ709 A498m]

RC889.A514   616.6'92   76–50145

ISBN 0–7216–1214–8

The endsheets are a composite of the infants born to couples who
were treated successfully for infertility by the authors.

Male Infertility   ISBN   0-7216-1214-8

Last digit is the print number: 9   8   7   6   5   4   3   2   1

To

DR. ROBERT S. HOTCHKISS

An inspiring teacher and pioneer
in the field of male infertility,
in recognition of his splendid
contributions to the plight of
the infertile couple.

FOREWORD

Finding an effective solution to the problem of a barren marriage has been a challenge to the physician since the beginning of history. Management of the infertile male has been a particular cause of frustration, especially in recent years. Patients have been frustrated because of the threat to their masculinity, the embarrassment of the necessary diagnostic studies, and the generally poor results of therapy. Urologists have been equally frustrated, and with good reason. In general, they have had a poor understanding of the field, and their attempts at diagnosis and treatment have been unrewarding. Semen analysis is as onorous to the urologist as routine blood counts are to the medical student. Until very recently, the urologist's diagnostic efforts revealed relatively few conditions that required surgical correction. Most urologists have thus neglected patients with problems related to infertility, concentrating instead on other conditions which seem more intellectually or financially rewarding.

The net result has been a generally inadequate service both to the patients and to their referring physicians. The need for such service was eloquently expressed by one of our colleagues, the late Dr. Sophia Kleegman, who said, "Infertility patients are not sick, but they are heartsick, and the help they seek is to them as urgent as any in medical practice." The American Board of Obstetrics and Gynecology has been concerned about this lack of professional support, and therefore has included male as well as female infertility in the new subspecialty division of Reproductive Endocrinology. Still another specialty, Andrology, is in its early phase of development. Clearly, if we urologists continue to do nothing to solve the problem, physicians in other disciplines certainly will.

Yet the problem is far from insoluble. As demonstrated in this book, recent research has led to a far better understanding of basic male reproductive physiology and a much greater knowledge of many of the causes of male infertility. The discovery and synthesis of hypothalamic-releasing factors and the development of more sophisticated biochemical methods of demonstrating the function of Leydig cells, germinal epithelium, and epididymis are examples of areas in which our knowledge is rapidly expanding. Several laboratories in university urology programs are now actively engaged in this type of research, and practical results are already beginning to emerge. Just as research in female reproduction several decades ago led to better understanding and methods of treatment of gynecologic problems, a more complete understanding of the basic physiology of male reproduction will undoubtedly lead to better methods of diagnosis and treatment of male infertility.

The evidence in this text shows that a definitive diagnosis can be made in most of these men. In my own view, the work-up of such patients can be done expeditiously and with reasonable accuracy by any practicing urologist. A pertinent history and limited physical examination, combined with appropriate laboratory tests, do not require an unreasonable amount of time. Routine semen analysis can easily be done by well-trained laboratory technicians; techniques of semen cytology are well established and most hospital pathologists can be of great help in developing accurate procedures for semen cytology. Indeed, seminal cytology correlates well with the cellular patterns seen on testicular biopsy and can be of considerable interest to the staff and residents in pathology as well as those in urology.

Equally important is the fact that at least 25 per cent of infertile men are found to have a surgically correctable varicocele, and over half of the patients father children after ligation of the internal spermatic vein. Perhaps another 10 per cent of patients require biopsy of the testis or vasography or both to determine the cause of severe oligospermia or azoospermia. Some of these patients eventually require surgery for the correction of ductal obstruction; the recent increase of patients requesting vasovasostomy after prior vasectomy adds significantly to the caseload of patients requiring reconstructive surgery for infertility. Finally, there are patients with epispadias, hypospadias, congenital chordee, and cryptorchism who require operative intervention to restore the potential for future fatherhood. Thus, when viewed in proper perspective, the segment of urology dealing with infertility is actually an active surgical practice, and need not be considered a basically medical subspecialty beneath the dignity of the urologist who enjoys the technical aspects of major surgery. Indeed, some of the most fascinating challenges to the active surgeon in the future may well lie in the area of microvascular repair of abnormalities of the vas, epididymis, and cord structures.

There has long been a need for a comprehensive compendium that includes the basic physiology of male reproduction, a practical yet complete modus operandi for the diagnostic study of infertile men, and a summary of the latest methods of therapy in this field. Doctors Amelar, Dubin, and Walsh have admirably accomplished this goal in this new work, which should be a part of the library of every practicing urologist. It is to be hoped that careful scrutiny of the material presented herein will not only increase the professional competence of surgeons in our field but also stimulate work that will lead to new knowledge and more effective methods of treatment of patients with the commonly occurring problem of a childless marriage.

BRUCE H. STEWART, M.D.

PREFACE

It is now estimated that in the United States, 15 per cent of marriages are involuntarily childless and another 10 per cent of couples have fewer children than they desire. The husband has been found to be the significant factor in about 30 per cent of these cases of infertility and to play an important contributing role in another 20 per cent. It is obvious that no evaluation of a barren marriage can be complete without a thorough evaluation of the male factor. The physician is therefore confronted with the problem of assessing the husband's role in the infertile marriage and determining what measures can be taken to treat the infertile husband.

A man must be capable of producing an adequate number of normal mature spermatozoa in his testicles to be considered fertile. These sperm cells are then transported through the epididymides and vasa deferentia, where they undergo further maturation and acquire the capacity for normal motility. The sperm are stored in the tails of the epididymides and in the ampullary portions of the vasa. The man must be capable of ejaculation, at which time the sperm are joined by the fluid products of the seminal vesicles and prostate. The ejaculum must pass outward through the urethral meatus and be deposited within the vagina at the appropriate time during the female cycle so that the sperm may migrate through the vaginal and cervical secretions and ascend through the uterus to the fallopian tubes and there fertilize the ovum.

There is now evidence that the process of sperm maturation is not halted at ejaculation but continues in the female reproductive tract, where the sperm cells undergo a definite change known as capacitation before becoming capable of penetrating the zona pellucida of the egg surface.

The purpose of this book is to serve as a practical guide for the diagnosis and therapy of male infertility. It is also a compendium of the basic physiology and pathophysiology of male reproduction which will provide the necessary background for rational therapy. This book should dispel the attitude that little or nothing can be done to improve the chances of fatherhood in the infertile man. The physician's use of these diagnostic and therapeutic measures will be rewarded by a higher rate of successful pregnancies than has even been thought possible by skeptics who regard the treatment of the infertile man as hopeless.

There must be a keen appreciation of the fact that reproduction involves the couple functioning together. Close cooperation between the family physician, the gynecologist, the urologist, the endocrinologist and the basic scientist is essential, and therapy requires a unified and compassionate approach to the problem of the infertile couple.

It is only recently that there has been full recognition and acceptance of the fact that the husband is frequently the cause for a couple's infertility. It is obvious to us as teachers that there is still a great need to educate clinicians and basic scientists regarding the magnitude of this problem. It is hoped that more investigators will study the problem with all of the scientific tools at their command. We must revise the curricula in our medical schools to emphasize the teaching of reproductive medicine and stimulate greater interest in this subject in the formative years in medical school and residency. Medical students and residents should also be exposed to private practice settings where reproductive problems are encountered.

RICHARD D. AMELAR, M.D.

LAWRENCE DUBIN, M.D.

PATRICK C. WALSH, M.D.

ACKNOWLEDGMENTS

We are grateful to Dr. Bruce Stewart, Attending Urologist at the Cleveland Clinic Foundation, for his warm friendship and encouragement. He served as the catalyst for this book by bringing us together to participate in seminars and postgraduate courses which he organized for the American Fertility Society and the American Urological Association. He stimulated and fostered our collaboration in producing this volume.

We are especially indebted to Cy Schoenfeld, Ph.D., Research Assistant Professor of Urology at New York University School of Medicine and Research Director of Fertility Laboratory, Inc. in New York City, for his careful review and contributions to the chapter on semen analysis, including the photomicrographs of the normal and abnormal sperm cells in this chapter. Dr. Schoenfeld's photography also illustrates the chapter on testicular biopsy.

Dr. Kurt Hirschhorn, Professor of Pediatrics and Genetics at Mount Sinai Medical School, and Jerome K. Sherman, Ph.D., Professor of Anatomy at the University of Arkansas School of Medicine, reviewed and updated sections of the chapter on artificial donor insemination.

The material on the legal aspects of donor insemination was brought up to date by Mrs. Harriet Pilpel and her colleague Mrs. Eva Paul, who are connected with the law firm of Greenbaum, Wolff and Ernst in New York City and have written and lectured extensively on artificial insemination and related subjects.

Mr. Neil O. Hardy, medical artist, supplied the drawings for Chapters 8 and 11.

We are most indebted to our diligent Editor, Mr. Brian Decker, who guided and encouraged us from the start.

Our secretary, Mrs. Shirley Sharpe, typed the manuscript.

Last but not least, we record our gratitude to our wives and children for their encouragement and patience.

RICHARD D. AMELAR, M.D.

LAWRENCE DUBIN, M.D.

PATRICK C. WALSH, M.D.

CONTENTS

Part I

PHYSIOLOGY AND PATHOPHYSIOLOGY OF THE MALE REPRODUCTIVE SYSTEM

Chapter 1

EMBRYOLOGY, ANATOMY, AND PHYSIOLOGY OF THE MALE REPRODUCTIVE SYSTEM

Patrick C. Walsh, M.D.
Richard D. Amelar, M.D.

EMBRYOLOGY OF THE MALE REPRODUCTIVE TRACT

Normal male sexual differentiation can be divided into early and late phases. During the early phase, which occurs during the first trimester, there is development of the definitive testis, the internal duct structures,

3

and the external genitalia. In the late phase during the second and third trimesters, there is growth of the external genitalia and descent of the testes. A complete understanding of the progression of these normal events is essential before the pathophysiology of abnormalities of sexual differentiation can be appreciated.

EARLY PHASE

The early phase of sexual differentiation is the result of a series of individual steps that occur in an orderly fashion (Table 1–1). Chromosomal factors direct the differentiation of the indifferent gonad into either an ovary or a testis. Then the fetal testis, acting via hormones, is responsible for differentiation of the internal ducts and the external genitalia. Consequently, three separate events occur in the early phase of sexual differentiation: differentiation of the testis, development of the internal ducts, and differentiation of the external genitalia.

Differentiation of the Testis

The first event in the differentiation of the testis, which occurs between the third and fifth week of gestation, is the formation of an indifferent gonad.[31] This gonadal primordium is composed of three cell types: (1) cells arising from the coelomic epithelium that form longitudinal folds on either side of the mesentery (genital ridges); (2) primordial germ cells that arise outside the urogenital ridge in the dorsal endodern of the yolk sac and migrate via the mesentery of the gut into the primitive gonad; and (3) mesenchymal cells that penetrate into the genital ridge from the adjacent mesonephros. Further development of this indifferent gonad into either an ovary or a testis is directed by chromosomal factors. In the male, beginning at 6 weeks of gestation, the primordial germ cells become incorporated into testicular cords. Later, at 9 weeks, Leydig cells are formed from the mesenchymal cells of the interstitium, and the surface germinal epithelium condenses to form the tunica albuginea. In the female, the indifferent gonad remains relatively unchanged until much later (13 to 16 weeks of gestation) when meiotic activity in the germ cells begins, follicles appear, and the ovarian stroma develops.

Until recently, it was thought that the Y chromosome was primarily responsible for directing testicular differentiation. This conclusion was based on early cytogenetic studies of patients with abnormalities of gonadal differentiation. Because 45/XO patients lacked a testis, and 47/XXY, 48/XXXY and 49 XXXXY patients developed testicular tissue, the Y chromosome appeared to bear the male determining factors. Likewise, it was assumed that two X chromosomes were necessary for normal ovarian differentiation. However, as more patients have been studied, new insight

Table 1-1 SUMMARY OF THE EARLY PHASE OF SEXUAL DIFFERENTIATION

PRIMORDIA	DETERMINANT	MALE DERIVATIVE	FEMALE DERIVATIVE	APPROXIMATE TIME (Weeks)
Indifferent gonad	Chromosomal XY XX	Testis	Ovary	6–8 15
Internal ducts	Fetal testicular secretion acting ipsilaterally			
Müllerian	Müllerian-inhibiting substance	Appendix testis	Fallopian tubes Uterus Upper vagina Gartner's duct	8–11
Wolffian	Testosterone	Epididymis Vas deferens Seminal vesicle		
Urogenital sinus and external genitalia				
Urogenital sinus	Dihydrotestosterone present (male)	Prostate Cowper's glands	Lower vagina Bartholin's glands Skene's glands	9–15
Genital tubercle		Glans penis	Clitoris	
Genital folds	Dihydrotestosterone absent (female)	Floor of penile urethra	Labia minor	
Genital swellings		Scrotum	Labia majora	

has been provided into the genetic factors responsible for normal gonadal development. These observations suggest that determinants on both the Y and X chromosome are necessary for normal testicular development.

The role of the Y chromosome in differentiation of the testis has recently been clarified. The exact location of the testis-determining gene on the Y chromosome is not certain, but presumably it is located on the short arm of the Y chromosome near the centromere. Recent studies have identified a locus of a histocompatibility antigen (H–Y antigen) that is linked so closely with the testis-determining gene that it may represent the testis-determining factor.[54] In the sex reversal syndrome, a condition in which phenotypic males have a 46/XX karyotype, small testes, azoospermia, and normal development of the external genitalia, the testes differentiate in the absence of a Y chromosome. Although the inheritance pattern in this syndrome suggests that an autosomal gene is involved in testicular differentiation in these individuals, it has recently been demonstrated that these patients are positive for the H–Y antigen.[75] Consequently, these data suggest that there has been translocation of the gene locus for the testis-determining factor from the short arm of the Y chromosome to an autosome. In the future, the measurement of the H–Y antigen will be important in studies of disorders of gonadal differentiation.

Evidence for X-chromosomal determinants directing testicular differentiation arises from studies of the syndrome of familial XY pure gonadal dysgenesis.[15] In this syndrome, phenotypic females with a 46/XY karyotype and bilateral streak gonads fail to develop a testis despite the presence of a Y chromosome. Because the inheritance in this syndrome appears to be X-linked, it is assumed that some determinant on the X chromosome is necessary for normal testicular development. Thus, it appears that factors on the X and Y chromosomes, and possibly also on autosomal chromosomes, are necessary for normal testicular differentiation.

Differentiation of Internal Ducts

Once the fetal testis is formed, it directs the differentiation of the internal ducts and the external genitalia. Prior to the onset of sexual differentiation, two sets of well-formed, primordial ducts are present in both male and female fetuses: the mesonephric or wolffian ducts, and the paramesonephric or müllerian ducts. The first event in the development of the male internal duct system is müllerian regression, which begins shortly after the onset of differentiation of the spermatic tubules of the testis. Although the cranial portion of each duct persists to form the appendix testis, and the extreme distal ends also remain, forming the prostatic utricle, the remainder of the müllerian duct disappears. Shortly thereafter, the proximal wolffian duct becomes elongated and convoluted, forming the epididymis, and the remainder of the duct gives rise to the vas deferens. At the extreme proximal end of the wolffian duct, the blind cranial end persists to form the appendix of the epididymis, and the adjacent portion connects with the seminiferous tubules to form the rete testis. At the caudal end of the wolffian duct, near its junction with the urogenital sinus, the vas becomes dilated, forming an ampulla from which a diverticulum arises to form the seminal vesicle. The portion of the duct between the seminal vesicle and the urethra becomes the ejaculatory duct.

Because the seminal vesicle is formed last, at approximately 13 weeks of gestation, it is possible to have a fully developed testis and epididymis with an underdeveloped vas deferens, seminal vesicle, and ejaculatory duct. If the entire vas deferens is undeveloped, a normal seminal vesicle or ejaculatory duct is impossible. If the mesonephric (wolffian) duct ceases development at a very early stage, the ureter and kidney will be absent on that side. As a practical point, when congenital absence of one kidney and ureter is suspected because of nonvisualization on an excretory urogram, inability to palpate a vas deferens in the scrotum on that side will confirm the diagnosis.[1]

In the female, the wolffian ducts regress and the müllerian ducts give rise to the fallopian tubes, the uterus, and the upper vagina. The development of the internal ducts is directed by the fetal testis, which secretes two hormones, androgen and müllerian-inhibiting substance.

Role of Fetal Testis.   The critical role of the fetal testis in directing differentiation of the internal ducts was first described by Jost.[30] In these experiments, rabbit embryos were castrated prior to the onset of sexual differentiation. In female embryos, castration did not interfere with differentiation of the internal ducts or the external genitalia. However, castration of male fetuses resulted in absence of wolffian duct structures, persistence of müllerian duct structures, and female differentiation of the urogenital sinus and external genitalia. These results indicated that the fetal testis was responsible for male phenotypic differentiation of the internal ducts and the external genitalia and that differentiation along female lines was entirely passive, occurring in the absence of a testis whether or not an ovary was present. Unilateral transplantation of a fetal testis into a female fetus caused unilateral regression of the müllerian duct and development of wolffian duct structures on that side. Implantation of a crystal of testosterone propionate into female rabbit fetuses produced extensive masculinization of the wolffian duct without inducing disappearance of the müllerian duct. These observations suggested that testosterone could not completely replace the fetal testicular secretion; consequently, it was deduced that two hormones from the fetal testis are essential for male development. One of these, an androgen, is responsible for virilization of the wolffian duct system to form the epididymis, vas deferens, and seminal vesicle and for virilization of the urogential sinus and external genitalia. The second hormone, called müllerian-inhibiting substance, is responsible for regression of the müllerian ducts in the male. In the presence of a fetal testis, müllerian-inhibiting substance produces regression of the müllerian duct and androgen

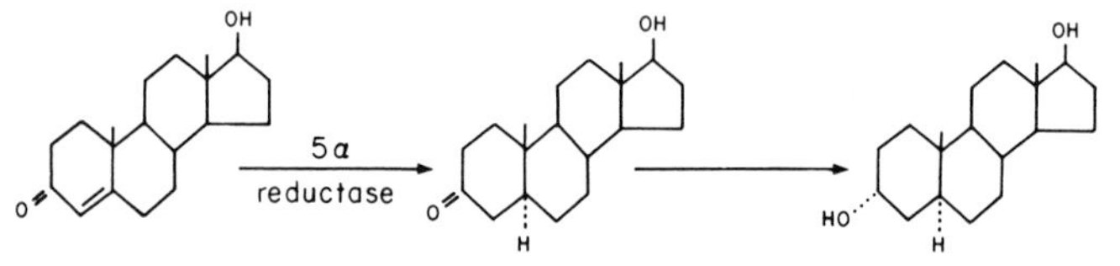

Testosterone   Dihydrotestosterone   Androstandiol
                          (5α–Androstan–17β ol–3 one)   (5α–Androstan–3α, 17β –diol .)

Figure 1–1.   Principal intracellular metabolic pathway to testosterone in the adult prostate and epididymis.

causes stimulation of the wolffian duct. In the absence of a fetal testis, as in the normal female, neither müllerian-inhibiting substance nor testosterone is secreted, and consequently the müllerian derivatives form and the wolffian ducts regress. It is important to recognize that these two secretions of the fetal testis act ipsilaterally.

Although the chemical nature of müllerian-inhibiting substance is not known for certain, it appears to be a polypeptide hormone that is secreted by the fetal Sertoli cells.[6] Much more is known about the androgen-dependent phases of sexual differentiation. Just prior to the onset of definitive male sexual differentiation, the fetal testis acquires the capacity to synthesize testosterone. At the same time, there is an increase in serum testosterone levels that peak at 11 to 17 weeks of fetal age and decline thereafter. Because the increase in serum testosterone concentration correlates with the peak in fetal human chorionic gonadotropin (HCG) concentrations, it seems reasonable to assume that during the critical stage of sexual differentiation in the male, the fetal Leydig cells are stimulated by chorionic gonadotropin.[12]

Effect of Testosterone.   The mechanism by which testosterone exerts its effect on differentiation of the wolffian ducts, urogenital sinus, and external genitalia has been carefully described by Wilson and co-workers.[65, 78] In postnatal life, accumulating evidence strongly suggests that testosterone must be converted to dihydrotestosterone by 5-α reductase enzymes located in target tissues, and that dihydrotestosterone is the active form of androgen in many target tissues, such as the prostate and epididymis, among others (Fig. 1–1). To determine whether dihydrotestosterone was also the androgen responsible for differentiation of the wolffian ducts, urogenital sinus, and external genitalia. Siiteri and Wilson examined various fetal tissues at the time of sexual differentiation to determine whether they were capable of converting testosterone to dihydrotestosterone.[65] Although the capacity to convert testosterone to dihydrotestosterone was present in the urogenital sinus and urogenital tubercle prior to the onset of male sexual differentiation, the capacity of the wolffian duct structures to form dihydrotestosterone did not develop until differentiation was far advanced. Accordingly, it was concluded that testosterone appears to be the intracellular mediator necessary for differentiation of the wolffian duct into the epididymis, the vas deferens, and the seminal vesicle, whereas dihydrotestosterone is the intracellular hormone responsible for virilization of the urogenital sinus and external genitalia. Supporting these conclusions is the fact that patients who lack the ability to form dihydrotestosterone (as in familial incomplete male pseudohermaphroditism, type II, also known as pseudovaginal perineoscrotal hypospadias) have a distinctive phenotype: the wolffian duct structures (epididymis, vas deferens, and seminal vesicles) are present, but the tissues derived from the urogenital sinus and from the anlage of the external genitalia are female in character.[76]

Differentiation of External Genitalia

Finally, development of the male external genitalia commences shortly after virilization of the wolffian duct. The urogenital sinus gives rise to the prostate, the genital tubercle forms the glans penis, the genital folds form the urethra and shaft of the penis, and the genital swellings merge and migrate inferiorly to form the scrotum. In the female, the urogenital sinus gives rise to the lower vagina, the genital tubercle forms the clitoris, the genital folds form the labia minora, and the genital swellings form the labia majora. As discussed previously, differentiation of the external genitalia and urogenital sinus is regulated by androgen. Testosterone, which is secreted into the systemic circulation, is converted to dihydrotestosterone by the $5\text{-}\alpha$ reductase enzymes located in the urogenital sinus and external genitalia.

LATE PHASE

When the early phase of sexual differentiation is completed, at the end of the first trimester of pregnancy, the testes are located at the level of the internal inguinal ring and the penis is only 3.5 mm. in length. At this age the penis in the male and the clitoris in the female are almost equal in size. Subsequently, during the last two trimesters of pregnancy, the size of the penis increases tenfold, i.e., from 3.5 to 35 mm. by the time of birth. The process of testicular descent remains dormant from the third to the seventh month of life, but during the last trimester the testes move from the internal ring through the inguinal canal into the scrotum. The mechanisms involved in this pase of testicular descent are uncertain, and a variety of theories have been proposed. At this time, the gubernaculum becomes swollen and the processus vaginalis grows very rapidly along the distended and swollen gubernaculum into the scrotal mesenchyme. Because of the swollen and distended gubernaculum, the diameters of the inguinal canal and the scrotum increase to the size of the testis or even larger. At that time, the testis descends because the degeneration of that part of the gubernaculum that is in contact with the epididymis and testis allows both structures to move along this hollowed-out path, first through the dilated inguinal canal and then into the scrotum. Although abdominal pressure may facilitate the passage of the testis from the abdomen through the internal ring, it is clear that endocrine factors play an important part in transinguinal migration of the testis. There is accumulating evidence that both gonadotropin and androgen are essential for growth of the penis and descent of the testis.

Although gonadotropin of placental origin appears to regulate the Leydig cell secretion of testosterone during the first trimester, there is other evidence suggesting that in the late phase of sexual differentiation (during the last two trimesters), which affects growth and development of the external genitalia and descent of the testes, the testes are under the regulation of the fetal pituitary gonadotropin. Kaplan et al. have demonstrated that the pituitary content of luteinizing hormone (LH) and follicle-stimulating hormone (FSH) and serum FSH levels are elevated in the second and third trimesters of pregnancy.[33] This occurs at a time when maternal HCG levels are falling. Because apituitary and anencephalic male fetuses frequently have undescended testes and hypoplasia of the penis and scrotum, it is assumed that during the second and third trimesters of pregnancy chorionic gonadotropin alone is generally insufficient to maintain adequate fetal Leydig cell function in the absence of FSH and LH secretion by the fetal pituitary.

DEVELOPMENT OF THE TESTES FROM BIRTH THROUGH PUBERTY

At birth, the testes are composed of small tubules filled with undifferentiated cells and a few spermatogonia. In addition, interstitial cells can be demonstrated, but they subsequently regress and are observed only rarely after 2 months of age. At term, a marked reduction in Leydig cell testosterone production has occurred, so that male and female cord serum testosterone concentrations are indistinguishable.[81] However, during the second week of life there is an abrupt increase in plasma testosterone levels, which reach a peak at 1 to 2 months of age with levels ranging from 53–360 ng./per 100 ml. By 6 months these levels have returned to baseline prepubertal levels (5 ng. per 100 ml.), where they remain until puberty. Presumably, this transient increase in plasma testosterone is due to abrupt elevations of serum LH and FSH that occur immediately after delivery.[80] By 4 months of age, serum LH and FSH levels have declined to the low levels characteristic of later childhood.

Between the ages of 4 and 10 years, the tubules slowly increase in tortuosity. Beginning at about age 10, the tubular epithelial cells increase in size and number, mitotic activity begins in the basally situated spermatogonia, primary and secondary spermatocytes and spermatids appear, and the undifferentiated cells mature into Sertoli cells. Thereafter, from approximately age 12, the tubules enlarge, Leydig cells mature, and the number of maturing tubules with active spermatogenesis increases.

The process of sexual maturation in which the sexually immature and infertile child is transformed into a sexually mature adolescent is known as puberty. Most of the visible changes that occur are due to the increased testicular secretion of testosterone in response to elevation of plasma gonadotropin levels (Fig. 1–2). Beginning at approximately age 6 to 8, there is an increase in serum FSH levels, and by age 10 to 12, mean serum FSH concentrations have entered the adult range. Luteinizing hormone increases at a slower rate until age 12, when there is a relatively greater increase in levels; the adult range is reached at approximately age 15 to 16. Along with this increase in serum LH levels there is an abrupt increase in blood testosterone beginning at approximately age 10 to 12 years and reaching a peak at age 16. This pattern of gonadotropin and plasma testosterone levels supports a model in which FSH plays a role primarily in testis growth and tubular development, and Leydig cell function depends primarily on LH.[79] In addition to the steady increase in serum LH levels that occurs throughout puberty, at midpuberty there is an increase in LH secretion at night that is associated with sleep.[7] This increase in LH secretory episodes corresponds to the number of sleep cycles of rapid and slow eye movements. In response to this increase in LH secretion, there is a corresponding elevation of plasma testosterone levels at night.[32] This increase in androgen could account for some of the early pubertal changes seen in males.

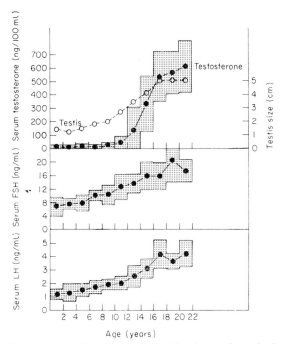

Figure 1–2. Cross sectional data demonstrating the changes in testis size and serum LH, FSH, and testosterone during sexual maturation in boys aged 2 to 21 years. (From Swerdloff, R. S., and Odell, W. D.: Postgrad. Med. J., *51*:200–208, 1975.)

The pubertal growth and maturation of the external genitalia and the pattern of pubic hair have been classified by Tanner into five stages.[48] His recommendations have been modified by Winter and Faiman to reduce interobserver variation.[79] Using their classification, the stages of pubertal development can be described as follows: P_1: prepubertal in all respects; mean length of testis less than 2.4 cm.; P_2: early testicular enlargement (2.4 to 3.2 cm. in longest diameter), sometimes associated with sparse hair at base of penis; P_3: long diameter of testis 3.3 to 4.0 cm., obvious pubic hair, beginning phallic enlargement, and possibly early axillary hair and gynecomastia or both; P_4: long diameter of testis 4.1 to 4.5 cm. adult amount of pubic hair, and moderate axillary hair; P_5: diameter of testis is over 4.5 cm., and adult secondary sexual characteristics are present. By utilizing these useful guidelines in examining prepubertal boys, the progression of sexual maturation can often be predicted. For example, if testicular length is greater than 2.4 cm. in the boy with delayed puberty, his parents can be reassured that pubertal development of the external genitalia is imminent. Genital development cannot be regarded as abnormally early if it begins after age 9 or unduly late if it begins before age 15.[48]

THE ADULT TESTIS

The adult testis normally measures 4.6 cm. in longest diameter (range 3.6 to 5.5 cm.) and 2.6 cm. in width (range 2.1 to 3.2 cm.) and weighs approximately 21 grams. The testis is surrounded by a thick white outer capsule composed of three layers: the visceral layer of the tunica vaginalis, the tunica albuginea, and the inner tunica vasculosa. The arterial blood supply to the testis arises from three sources: (1) the internal spermatic artery, which arises from the aorta; (2) the deferential or vasal artery, which arises from the hypogastric artery; and (3) the cremasteric artery. In man, the deferential and cremasteric arteries provide an important source of collateral circulation for the testis. In approximately a third of men, the sum of the diameters of these two arteries is at least equal to that of the diameter of the testicular artery.[23] The venous collaterals from the testis and epididymis join to form the pampiniform plexus, which drains via the internal spermatic vein into the inferior vena cava on the right and the renal vein on the left. The veins of the testis are superficial and lie close to the subcutaneous tissues of the scrotum so that the returning venous blood is very close to scrotal temperature.[20] Harrison and Weiner suggest that the intimate relationship of arteries and veins in the spermatic cord, coupled with the slow nonpulsatile blood flow in the spermatic artery, provides a mechanism for precooling arterial blood before it reaches the testis.[24] Experimental studies in several species have demonstrated that the blood within the internal spermatic arteries cools as it approaches the testis, losing heat to the adjacent venous system by countercurrent heat exchange.[20]

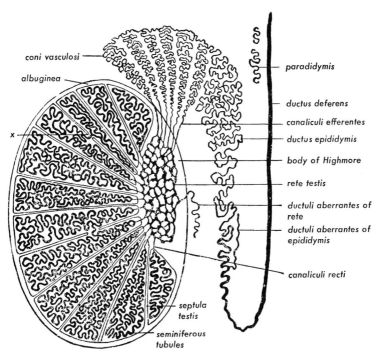

Figure 1–3. Diagram of arrangement of seminiferous tubules and excretory ducts in the testis and epididymis. (From Bloom, W., and Fawcett, D. W.: A Textbook of Histology, 10th ed. Philadelphia, W. B. Saunders Company, 1975.)

In man, the abdominoscrotal temperature difference averages approximately 2.2° C.

Beneath the white outer capsule of the testis, the seminiferous tubules are separated by fibrous septa into about 250 pyramidal lobules (Fig. 1–3). Each lobule contains several coiled, U-shaped seminiferous tubules, 30 to 60 cm. in length, with both ends terminating in straight tubules called canaliculi recti. These short straight tubules connect directly with the rete testis. Because the seminiferous tubules occupy over 75 per cent of the total mass of the testis, when isolated damage to the tubules occurs the testes become small and soft. The seminiferous tubules have a central lumen, a stratified epithelium four to eight cells in thickness composed of Sertoli cells and spermatogenic cells, and an outer thin basement membrane surrounded by a fibrous tunica propria (Fig. 1–4). The interstitial tissue between the tubules is compsed of Leydig cells, blood vessels, extensive lymphatic channels, and numerous macrophages.

SERTOLI CELLS

The Sertoli cells are tall columnar cells that extend radially from just within the basement membrane toward the lumen of the seminiferous tu-

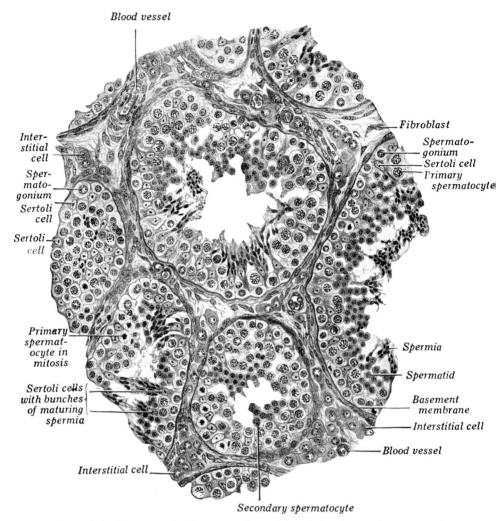

Blood vessel

Fibroblast

Inter-
stitial
cell

Spermato-
gonium

Sertoli cell

Sper-
mato-
gonium

Primary
spermatocyte

Sertoli
cell

Sertoli
cell

Primary
spermat-
ocyte in
mitosis

Spermia

Spermatid

Sertoli cells
with bunches
of maturing
spermia

Basement
membrane

Interstitial cell

Blood vessel

Interstitial cell

Secondary spermatocyte

Figure 1–4. Human testis. The transections of the tubules show various stages of spermatogenesis. 170 ×. (From Maximow, A. A., and Bloom, W.: A Textbook of Histology,
Philadelphia, W. B. Saunders Co., 1957.)

bules. Their cytoplasmic borders are indefinite, and frequently spermatocytes and spermatids can be seen embedded in their cytoplasm. Fawcett and
coworkers have demonstrated that the Sertoli cells are linked in tight junctions that divide the seminiferous tubule into two compartments: a basal
compartment, occupied by spermatogonia and preleptotene spermatocytes,
and an adluminal compartment containing more advanced stages of the
germ cell population (Fig. 1–5). Consequently, the seminiferous epithelium
is divided into a fixed population of supporting Sertoli cells and a mobile,
continuously escalating population of germ cells.[17] The exact functions of
the Sertoli cells have yet to be elucidated. Sertoli first suggested that these

supporting cells were "nursing cells" for the germinal epithelium. More recent evidence suggests that the Sertoli cell has several functions: maintenance of the blood-testis barrier; secretion of the testicular fluid and androgen-binding protein; and participation in the release of sperm.[17] Fawcett and co-workers have demonstrated that the tight junctions between adjacent Sertoli cells, in combination with the myoid cells of the peritubular contractile cell layer, are the anatomic structures that are the principal components of the blood-testis barrier. The Sertoli cells secrete fluid into the seminiferous tubules, thereby creating a micro-environment in the adluminal compartment of the seminiferous tubules that in some ways facilitates meiosis and spermiogenesis. One substance secreted by the Sertoli cell is a high affinity binding protein for testosterone and dihydrotestosterone.[21] The presence of this androgen-binding protein (ABP) in the seminiferous tubule may generate a diffusion potential that results in the inflow and

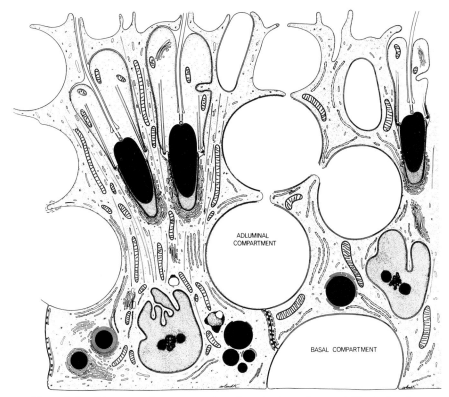

Figure 1–5. Diagrammatic representation of an electron micrograph illustrating the manner in which occluding junctions between Sertoli cells divide the seminiferous epithelium into a basal compartment occupied by the spermatogonia and preleptotene spermatocytes and an adluminal compartment containing more advanced stages of the germ-cell population. (From Fawcett, D. W.: *In* Greep, R. O., and Astwood, E. B. (eds.): Handbook of Physiology. Section 7, Vol. 5, Washington, D.C., Amer. Physiol. Soc., 1975.)

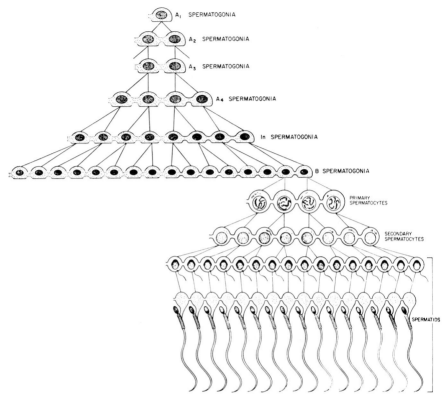

Figure 1–6. Diagram of the stages of spermatogenesis demonstrating the intracellular bridges that link adjacent developing germ cells. (From Dym, M., and Fawcett, D. W.: Further observations on the numbers of spermatogonia, spermatocytes and spermatids connected by intracellular bridges in the mammalian tests: Biol. Reprod., *4*:195, 1971.)

accumulation of androgen in the immediate environment of the germ cells. In addition, it may allow high concentrations of androgen to be transported via the testicular fluid to the caput epididymis. The secretion of this androgen-binding protein by the Sertoli cell appears to be regulated by testosterone and possibly FSH.[72]

GERMINAL EPITHELIUM

The spermatogenic cells are arranged in an orderly manner from the basement membrane to the lumen. Spermatogonia lie directly on the basement membrane, and next to them, progressing centrally, are found primary spermatocytes, secondary spermatocytes (rarely seen because they have a short half-life), and spermatids (Fig. 1–4). Within these broad groups at least 13 recognizable germ cell types have been identified in the human testis: dark type A spermatogonia (Ad); pale type A spermatogonia (Ap); type B spermatogonia (B); preleptotene primary spermatocytes (R); leptotene primary spermatocytes (L); zygotene primary spermatocytes (Z); pachytene primary spermatocytes (P); secondary spermatocytes (II); and spermatids Sa, Sb$_1$, Sc, Sd, and Sd$_2$.

In sperm maturation, the most primitive undifferentiated spermatogonia are the stem cells. In the process called stem cell renewal, these primitive cells must be constantly replenished. Clermont believes that when Ap spermatogonia undergo mitotic division, two populations of cells can be produced: (1) other type Ap spermatogonia that will replenish the stock of primitive stem cells, and (2) type B spermatogonia that will differentiate into spermatozoa.[13] Through a series of mitotic divisions, the type B spermatogonia differentiate into pachytene primary spermatocytes (Fig. 1–6). The primary spermatocytes undergo the first maturation division by a process of meiosis, giving rise to two secondary spermatocytes. Each secondary spermatocyte divides to form two spermatids, thereby reducing the number of chromosomes from 46 to 23. The spermatid does not undergo further division but matures into a spermatozoon. The time necessary to produce a spermatozoon from a pale type A spermatogonia is 74 days.[26]

LEYDIG CELLS

The Leydig cells are found in the loose connective tissue stroma between the tubules, usually in small groups of from 5 to 20 cells. The Leydig cells constitute about 12 per cent of the testicular volume and are the principal source of testosterone production, secreting approximately 7 mg. of testosterone per day.[41] Once testosterone is formed in the interstitial tissue, it leaves by the capillary venous or lymphatic route or by traversing the myoid cell layer to enter the seminiferous tubules.[11] In addition to testosterone, the human testis also secretes dihydrotestosterone, estradiol, estrone, pregnenolone, 17-hydroxypregnenolone, Δ5-androstanediol, 17-hydroxyprogesterone, and progesterone.[41] It is unclear whether the Leydig cell is the major source of these metabolites or whether they arise from cells in the seminiferous tubule.

HYPOTHALAMIC-PITUITARY AXIS

The testes are regulated by two pituitary gonadotropins: (1) luteinizing hormone (LH) or interstitial cell stimulating hormone, and (2) follicle-stimulating hormone (FSH). These hormones are synthesized and stored in the anterior pituitary and their release is regulated by centers in the hypothalamus. Until relatively recently it was believed that two neurohormonal substances, LH-releasing hormone and FSH-releasing hormone, were secreted into the hypothalamic-pituitary portal vascular system and regulated gonadotropin release. However, Schally and co-workers have isolated and synthesized a decapeptide, gonadotropin-releasing hormone (GnRH) that releases both LH and FSH.[61] When GnRH is administered intravenously to humans, it results in a prompt increase in serum LH and, to a much lesser extent, FSH levels in the blood. The response of the pituitary to GnRH is modulated by steroidal hormones. Estradiol inhibits the effects of GnRH on LH and FSH secretions.[60a]

LH and FSH, which are glycopeptides, are synthesized in the pituitary and are composed of two polypeptide chains: (1) the α-chain, which is the same for LH, FSH, and thyroid-stimulating hormone and (2) the β-chain, which provides for the biological specificity of the molecule. LH and FSH are secreted from the pituitary into the general circulation in an episodic fashion. This results in rhythmic elevations in serum LH levels that occur at 60- to 100-minute intervals and vary from 20 to 400 per cent.[53] Because the metabolic clearance rate of FSH is much slower than that for LH, the longer survival of FSH in the circulation is reflected by more constant serum levels of this hormone.

LH and FSH are transported to the systemic blood stream to the testes, where they exert their effect. LH acts on the Leydig cell to stimulate the secretion of testosterone. The biochemical events mediating this important effect have been well described.[9] LH binds to receptors located on the Leydig cell membrane, resulting in the activation of adenyl cyclase which in turn activates the conversion of adenosine triphosphate (ATP) to cyclic adenosine monophosphate (cAMP). By some as yet unidentified mechanism, this enhances the conversion of cholesterol to pregnenolone, thus providing more pregnenolone for conversion to testosterone. The effects of FSH are less certain. Utilizing the fluorescent antibody technique, FSH has been localized to the Sertoli cells. Means has demonstrated membrane receptors for FSH and FSH-induced activation of adenyl cyclase in membranes isolated from seminiferous tubules.[50] However, the exact role of FSH in the regulation of spermatogenesis is unclear.

ROLE OF GONADOTROPINS IN SPERMATOGENESIS

In discussing the role of gonadotropins in regulating spermatogenesis, a clear distinction must be drawn between the *initiation* and the *maintenance* of spermatogenesis. Initiation refers to stimulation of mature spermatogenesis in the prepubertal testis or in the testis with atrophic tubules after hypophysectomy. Maintenance of spermatogenesis refers to the necessary hormonal requirements once full spermatogenesis is present. In an excellent review, Steinberger summarized the experimental evidence of the hormonal requirements that are necessary for the *initiation* of spermatogenesis.[69] He stated that hormones are not required for the formation of type A and B spermatogonia, for the formation of primary spermatocytes, or for the progression of the meiotic prophase. However, for the differentiation of late primary (pachytene) spermatocytes to mature spermatozoa, two hormones act sequentially: testosterone (synthesized by the Leydig cells under the regulation of LH) and FSH. Testosterone acts first to stimulate primary spermatocytes to complete the meiotic division with the formation of secondary spermatocytes and young spermatids. Testosterone must be present in high local concentrations to exert this influence. Such concentrations are possible owing to the anatomic location of the Leydig cell just a few microns from the germinal epithelium. Finally, FSH acts to induce maturation of late spermatids to mature spermatozoa. Once spermatogenesis is initiated, it is unclear whether or not FSH is necessary for the *maintenance* of spermatogenesis. The evidence for this is based on a number of experimental observations. Following hypophysectomy in rats, if immediate treatment with testosterone in large doses or with LH is given, spermatogenesis is maintained without the addition of FSH.[14, 66] If testicular atrophy is permitted to occur after hypophysectomy, then both LH and FSH are necessary for the initiation of spermatogenesis. However, once spermatogenesis is established, therapy with LH alone will sustain the production of mature sperm. MacLeod has documented this effect of LH in humans.[43] Recently, Sherins *et al.* have demonstrated that in the majority of men receiving HCG for long periods of time, spermatogenesis is maintained despite the reduction of circulating FSH to levels that are too low to be measured.[63] In this study, as in the hypophysectomy experiments in which complete removal of the pituitary was uncertain, it is possible that permissive amounts of FSH were present. However, these studies do seriously challenge the central role of FSH as the primary regulator of spermatogenesis.

The hypothalamic-pituitary-gonadal system consists of a closed-loop feedback control mechanism directed at maintaining normal reproductive functions. In this manner, hormones produced by the testes have inhibitory effects on the secretion of LH and FSH. Although it is generally accepted that testosterone is the principal feedback regulator of LH release, the substance responsible for the feedback regulation of FSH remains poorly understood. Castration results in an elevation of both LH and FSH. However, selective germ cell damage (produced by heat, irradiation, or chemotherapy) that leaves Leydig cell function undisturbed produces an elevation of serum FSH but not LH. Consequently, it has been suggested that the testis produces two hormones, one of which is a product of spermatogenic tissue. McCullagh named this substance inhibin,[49] and Johnsen subsequently suggested that it was a lipid found in the residual bodies split off from spermatozoa.[29] Other studies indicated that it was nonsteroidal and water-soluble. Howard suggested that this substance was an estrogen secreted by the Sertoli cell.[27] Lacy, combined the inhibin theory with the observation that residual bodies are phagocytized by the Sertoli cells, suggest that the residual bodies provide the substrate for the production of estrogen.[38] More recent evidence suggests that the cell involved in the regulation of FSH must be either the type A spermatogonium or the Sertoli cell.[51]

Recent studies have clarified the role of steroidal hormones in the feedback regulation of FSH. Studies in both the rat and humans have demonstrated that testosterone and estradiol influence both FSH and LH secretions.[39, 64, 71, 77] However, neither steroid preferentially suppresses FSH. In the rat, Swerdloff et al. have tested a wide range of C_{18}, C_{19}, and C_{21} steroids and again have failed to identify any agent that selectively inhibits FSH.[70] These data suggest that although estradiol and testosterone may have an important role in FSH feedback control, they affect FSH and LH in a parallel fashion. There appears to be another factor with selective or preferential effects on the inhibition of FSH secretion. Baker et al. have recently summarized the evidence for the presence of a water-soluble, nonsteroidal substance that is present in the rete testis fluid and selectively suppresses FSH.[3]

EPIDIDYMIS

The testicular spermatozoa undergo anatomic, biochemical, and functional changes as they pass through the epididymis. In this capacity, the epididymis provides transport, maturation, and storage of spermatozoa. From the seminiferous tubule, testicular spermatozoa and secretions travel to the rete testis; from there they move into the efferent ductule and then into the epididymis. The epididymis is a single, highly convoluted duct 4 to 5 meters in length that can be divided into three regions: the caput, the corpus, and the cauda. It is important to recognize that the epididymis is composed of a single duct, and consequently inadvertent injury to the epididymis (e.g., in the process of testicular biopsy) will produce total obstruction. The arterial blood supply to the epididymis is derived from the testicular, epididymal, vasal, and cremasteric arteries. The autonomic nerve supply arises from the intermediate and inferior spermatic nerves, which arise from the superior portion of the hypogastric plexus and from the vesical plexus respectively. Testicular spermatozoa are transported to the epididymis by secretions from the testis and by ciliary and contractile activity of the luminal wall of the efferent ductules. In the epididymis, regular contractions of the ductile wall appear to provide the motile force for the transport of spermatozoa from the caput to the cauda.[5] In humans, the mean epididymal transit time is approximately 12 days.[60]

The two major functions of the epididymis are maturation of the spermatozoa and storage. It is well known that testicular spermatozoa lack motility and fertilizing capacity. However, in the epididymis important maturational changes occur. For example, Orgebin-Crist demonstrated that spermatozoa collected from the caput, corpus, and cauda epididymidis fertilized 1 per cent, 63 per cent and 92 per cent of exposed oocytes respectively.[55] As summarized by Bedford, the alteration in the functional state of epididymal spermatozoa may be reflected in: (1) development of the capacity for sustained progressive motility; (2) modification of the metabolic character and the structural state of certain tail organelles and of sperm nuclear chromatin; (3) alteration of the surface of the plasma membrane; (4) morphologic changes involving movement and loss of the middle-piece remnant of the spermatid cytoplasm (cytoplasmic droplets); and (5) modification of the form of the acrosome.[5] Once these maturational events have occurred, the spermatozoa are transported from the proximal part of the epididymis to the cauda by mild autonomous peristaltic contractions of the wall of the duct. There the spermatozoa may be retained and stored in a functional state for several weeks.

The structural and functional integrity of the epididymis, the acquisition of fertilizing capacity by spermatozoa, and the viability of spermatozoa within the epididymis are all androgen-dependent processes. Castration, hypophysectomy, or treatment with antiandrogens markedly affects these processes.[56] Testosterone in high concentration (approximately 20-fold greater than plasma levels) is transported bound to the high affinity androgen-binding protein from the seminiferous tubules via rete testis fluid into the epididymis.[21] In the epididymis, the androgen-binding protein disappears, and testosterone is taken up by the epididymal cells and converted to 5α-dihydrotestosterone and 5α-androstane-3α,17 β-diol (Fig. 1–1). These androgens appear to be essential for the development of fertilizing capacity of epididymal spermatozoa.[42]

VAS DEFERENS

The vas deferens is easily palpable in the scrotum as a portion of the spermatic cord. It is about 35 cm. in length and extends from the cauda epididymis through the external and internal inguinal rings and then over the ureter and behind the bladder. The terminal section enlarges to form an ampullary portion that joins the duct of the seminal vesicle, forming the ejaculatory duct. Histologically, the vas deferens is lined by mucosa and is surrounded by a wall composed of three layers of smooth muscle: longitudinal muscle in the outer and inner layers and circular muscle in the middle. This muscular wall afford powerful peristaltic motion. Exterior to this muscle layer there is a thick sheath of connective tissue. The epithelial lining of the lumen varies along the length of the vas deferens.[73] Near the epididymis the mucosa resembles the epithelium in the cauda epididymidis and is characterized by large columnar cells with regularly placed pairs of cilia that are actually stereocilia or microvilli that may have an absorptive

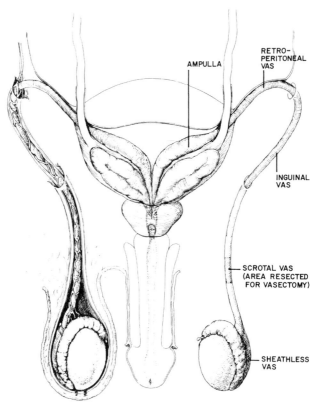

Figure 1–7. The five portions of the vas deferens. (From Hulka, J. F., and Davis, J. F.: Vasectomy and reversible vasocclusion. Fertil. Steril., *23*:684, 1972.)

function.[57] These stereocilia do not move as do the cilia of the rete testis and the efferent ductules. Distally, the epithelial cells lining the lumen of the vas deferens become nonciliated and smaller in size.

Anatomically the vas deferens may be divided into five portions: (1) the sheathless epididymal portion contained within the tunica vaginalis; (2) the scrotal portion; (3) the inguinal portion; (4) the retroperitoneal or pelvic portion; and (5) the ampulla (Fig. 1–7). The portion of the vas deferens of clinical interest for performing vasectomy is generally in the midscrotal portion.

The blood supply to the vas deferens is derived from the deferential artery, a branch of the inferior vesical artery, which provides an important collateral blood supply to the testis. At the time of vasectomy, if the deferential artery is not carefully ligated or coagulated it may be a potential site of hemorrhage. The sheath of the vas deferens contains nerve fibers for pain and sympathetic fibers that release norepinephrine.[74] These fibers may be responsible for the presence of the spontaneous motility of the human vas deferens that has been demonstrated *in vitro*. The presence of spontaneous motility *in vitro* leads to the working hypothesis that there is spontaneous motility of the human vas deferens *in vivo*. Tone in the sympathetic fibers innervating the vas deferens is probably dependent on the integrity of the spinal center. It is believed that the intrinsic rhythmicity of the vas deferens depends upon the local concentration of norepinephrine. However, the powerful and coordinated series of contractions that propel sperm from the epididymis to the urethra during ejaculation are initiated and controlled by the release of substantial amounts of norepinephrine from the sympathetic nerve endings. It is well known that spermatozoa are expelled from the cauda epididymidis and vas deferens at the time of ejaculation. Utilizing radiographic cinematography techniques. Mitsuya *et al.* have demonstrated this by injecting radiographic media into the vas deferens prior to ejaculation.[52]

Vasectomy results in the division of the inferior spermatic nerve that runs parallel to the vas deferens and innervates it. Attempts at vasectomy reversal may fail to restore fertility because, although the sympathetic fibers are strongly regenerative and consequently if divided would probably grow from the vas deferens to reinnervate the lower vas and epididymis, iatrogenic surgical factors may prevent regeneration and restoration of the sympathetic nerve supply. These factors include: (1) the removal of a large segment of the vas; (2) the placement of a suture or clip too close to the sheath around the stump of the vas; and (3) an inflammatory reaction in scar tissue in response to the trauma of the operation.[28] An intact sympathetic nerve supply is probably essential for the transport of sperm from the epididymis at the time of ejaculation. Without such a supply to the vas deferens and epididymis, complete recovery of sperm output is unlikely to be achieved after a functional vasovasostomy.

Leiter and Brendler first noted that aspermia, or failure of any ejaculate to appear at the time of orgasm, may be due to neurogenic causes.[40] In 1968, Girgis *et al.* discovered that 7 out of 49 of their patients actually had complete absence of ejaculation due to neurogenic causes rather than retrograde ejaculation as had been previously supposed.[18] This type of aspermia may be temporary, as in chemical sympathectomy, or permanent, as in surgical sympathectomy. Kom *et al.* confirmed this finding in 1971, reporting a loss of emission rather than retrograde ejaculation after retroperitoneal lymphadenectomy.[36] They atrributed this to resection of the lumbar sympathetic chain. Most recently, Kedia *et al.*, in a study of 40 patients who underwent retroperitoneal lymph node dissection for the treatment of testicular tumors, observed that although the patients were potent and were capable of the sensation of ejaculation, there was no seminal emission.[34] They suggested that the failure of ejaculation in these patients was due to absent contraction of the seminal vesicles and vasa deferentia rather than retrograde ejaculation. as had been previously thought. They also found that men treated with sympatholytic drugs, such as guanethidine, experience the same phenomenon — normal erections and orgasms but no ejaculation.

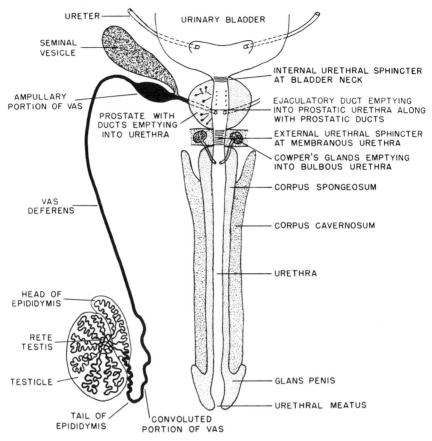

Figure 1–8. Schematic representation of the male genital organs, illustrating the relation of the prostate and ejaculatory ducts to the internal and external sphincters, bladder, and urethra. (From Amelar, R. D.: Infertility in Men. Philadelphia, F. A. Davis Co., 1966.)

SEMINAL VESICLES AND PROSTATE

The seminal vesicles are paired, elongated glands that were so-named because of the erroneous notion that they were reservoirs for semen. They provide a source of nutrient fructose and a proteinaceous material that contains a substrate for the enzymatic process of seminal coagulation. The prostate, which is approximately the size of a chestnut, is a firm, elastic tubuloalveolar gland that surrounds the urethra immediately below the bladder neck. It is pierced by the ejaculatory ducts that enter the urethra midway between the internal urethral sphincter at the bladder neck and the external urethral sphincter at the urogenital diaphragm (Fig. 1–8).

Human seminal plasma is composed of fluids secreted by the prostate, seminal vesicles, bulbourethral (Cowper's) glands, urethral (Littre's) glands, and the scant fluid from the epididymides and testes. The prostatic secretion contributes 13 to 32 per cent of the ejaculate, and the seminal vesicles provide the major portion of the seminal plasma, from 46 to 80 per cent.[8] At ejaculation, spermatozoa are mixed with these secretions. Only a small portion of the seminal fluid is actually composed of sperm cells, perhaps less than 0.1 per cent by volume.

The seminal plasma of the human ejaculate usually amounts to 3 or 4 ml. Among its characteristic chemical constituents are choline, spermine, various carbohydrates and organic acids, numerous proteins and peptides, free amino acids, and a number of highly active enzymes.[47] In addition, there are at least 13 prostaglandins. These substances were first noted in the seminal plasma in 1931 by Kurzok and Lieb.[37] They noted that if a strip of human uterus is suspended in a 100-ml. bath to which 1 ml. of human seminal plasma is added, there follows an increase and then a decrease in the spontaneous contractions of the uterine muscle. Shortly thereafter, Euler in Sweden concluded that the uterus-stimulating activity of seminal plasma came from a prostaglandin that he isolated and purified.[16] Although initially it was thought that this substance was of prostatic origin, it is now clear that prostaglandins are derived from the seminal vesicle. The major prostaglandins in human seminal plasma include prostaglandin (PG) E_1, PGE_2, PGE_3, PGF_1, and PGF_2. PGE_1 and PGE_2 together constitute about 5 mg per 100 ml. of semen.[47] All of the other prostaglandins together also contribute approximately 5 mg. per 100 ml.

In the contractions during the process of ejaculation, the exact role of neither the prostaglandins nor the various biogenic amines (such as norepinephrine, histamine, acetylcholine, and serotonin) has been clearly explained. In man, the contractions are thought to begin in Cowper's glands and extend subsequently to the prostate and the ampullae of the vasa deferentia, and lastly to the seminal vesicles.[46] Disturbances in these contractions can be induced by drugs such as reserpine, amphetamine, and chlorpromazine, all of which can produce a complete reversal of the ejaculatory sequence.[45] Amelar and Hotchkiss reported that a reversal of the ejaculatory process occurs normally in 6 per cent of infertile men.[2]

In addition to the prostaglandins, the seminal plasma contains various other fatty acids and a wide range of organic acids such as citric, ascorbic, and lactic acids.[47] The major carbohydrate in seminal plasma is fructose, but there are also small amounts of sorbitol and inositol, glucose, ribose, fucose, and trace amounts of several other sugars. The seminal plasma contains several specific proteins, including some that undergo coagulation at the time of ejaculation.

The occurrence in the seminal plasma of many unusual and often unique substances in amounts often exceeding those that exist elsewhere in the body has led to much speculation about their possible role in reproductive physiology. Although much is known of the chemistry of the seminal plasma and its effects on spermatozoa *in vitro*,[44, 46] the physiologic importance of these substances *in vivo* is not well understood. It is highly likely that spermatozoa remain in contact with the seminal plasma for only a short time.[67]

Infertile patients with azoospermia due to congenital bilateral absence of the vasa deferentia are not as rare as previously suspected. Indeed, this condition has been found to be the cause of infertility in 152 (2 per cent) of 7600 patients examined by Amelar and Dubin since 1956. These patients have scant ejaculate volumes because the seminal vesicles are also congenitally absent. Their ejaculate therefore does not contain fructose, and because the substrate for seminal coagulum formation also originates in the seminal vesicles, their semen does not coagulate immediately after ejaculation. When the vasa deferentia cannot be palpated in the scrotum, these simple observations of the semen of azoospermic patients with low semen volume will confirm the diagnosis without the necessity for surgical scrotal exploration.

EJACULATION

Observations of the semen have demonstrated that the distribution of the sperm cells is not uniform throughout the ejaculatory process. This conclusion has been arrived at by using the split ejaculate method, in which the total seminal specimen is partitioned or fractionated during the ejaculatory process, the various fractions then being examined separately[2] (see Chapter 5). In man, the different portions of the semen usually follow one another in a definite sequence. It is known that during ejaculation the three main glandular systems that contribute to the ejaculate discharge successively. Ejaculation begins with the scant secretions of Cowper's glands, followed immediately by secretions from the prostate, which contain the main bulk of acid phosphatase. This secretion is joined by material which has accumulated within the ampullary portion of the vas deferens, composed of products from the testes, the epididymides, and the vasa deferentia. Consequently, this portion contains the highest concentration of spermatozoa. The last portion contains the highest concentration of fructose, the substance specific to the seminal vesicles. The products of these three systems become more or less mixed during ejaculation. Collection of the ejaculate in separate fractions and subsequent estimation of the amount of acid phosphatase, spermatozoa, and fructose in each fraction make it possible to calculate the amount contributed by each component of the reproductive system.

If during the collection of the semen specimen the ejaculate is divided into two containers, it will be found that there are significant differences between the first and second portions with regard to viscosity, sperm concentration, sperm motility, and sperm morphology. Compared to the total ejaculate, these differences may be profound. The use of the split ejaculate in the management of male infertility is discussed in Chapter 10.

The ejaculatory ducts empty into the urethra between the internal and external urethral sphincters (Fig. 1–8). Normally, during the process of ejaculation reflex closure of the bladder neck and relaxation of the external sphincter occur, forcing the ejaculate toward the urethral meatus. These reflexes are mediated by sensory nerves from the prostatic urethra that excite centers in the sacral and lumbar regions of the spinal cord. These nerves in turn transmit impulses over autonomic and somatic pathways. Sympathetic stimulation results in contraction of the internal sphincter at the vesical neck, preventing retrograde passage of semen into the bladder.[58] The external sphincter is actively relaxed by parasympathetic activity. Somatic nerves cause contraction of the striated bulbocavernosus muscle.

Retrograde ejaculation of semen into the urinary bladder may occur following disruption of the internal sphincter by transurethral or open resection or prostatic or bladder neck tissue. It may also occur in some diabetic males due to diabetic neuropathy,[19] after lumbar sympathectomy,[59] following treatment with drugs that interfere with the local release of norepinephrine from the sympathetic nerve terminals (e.g., guanethidine),[62] after spinal cord injury,[68] or after combined abdominoperineal resection of the colon and rectum. A new type of retrograde ejaculation was recently reported in three men who had low semen volume (0.3 to 0.6 ml.), absence of fructose in the seminal fluid, and azoospermia.[35] They all had palpable vasa deferentia, and large numbers of apparently normal sperm were found in the urinary bladder after retrograde ejaculation.

CAPACITATION

There is evidence that the process of sperm maturation is not halted at ejaculation but continues in the female reproductive tract, where the spermatozoa undergo a definite change known as capacitation before becoming capable of penetrating the zona pellucida of the ovum. The nature of capacitation is unknown, but most authorities agree that it is a necessary prerequisite to fertilization in man.[10] Capacitation may represent a final stage of sperm maturation, possibly involving removal or neutralization of a protective coating from the sperm surface that was acquired in the epididymis or upper reaches of the male reproductive tract.[10]

It has been demonstrated that human sperm survive in a state of motility for a maximum of 90 hours within the female genital tract. Although it is unknown how long spermatozoa remain fertile in the female genital tract, it has been concluded from experimental observations in eight animal species that spermatozoa lose their ability to fertilize in approximately half the time that motility is extinguished. Thus, it is estimated that the maximal functional survival time of human spermatozoa within the female genital tract is less than 48 hours. Since the human ovum has a maximal survival time of 1 day, the fertile period for any human female cycle is about 3 days.[25]

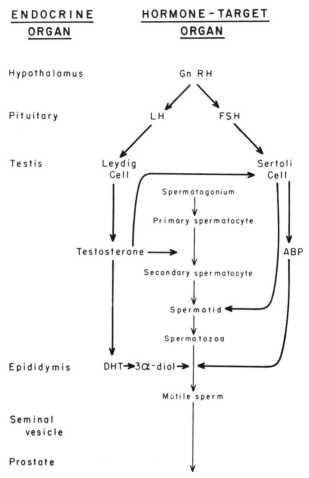

ENDOCRINE ORGAN

HORMONE-TARGET ORGAN

Hypothalamus — Gn RH

Pituitary — LH   FSH

Testis — Leydig Cell   Sertoli Cell

Spermatogonium

Primary spermatocyte

Testosterone

Secondary spermatocyte   ABP

Spermatid

Spermatozoa

Epididymis — DHT→3α-diol→

Motile sperm

Seminal vesicle

Prostate

Figure 1–9. Schematic summary of the hormonal regulation of reproductive function in men. Gonadotropin-releasing hormone (GnRH); luteinizing hormone (LH); follicle-stimulating hormone (FSH); androgen-binding protein (ABP); dihydrotestosterone (DHT); 3α-andro-stanediol (3α-diol).

SUMMARY

In schematic form, Figure 1–9 summarizes the hormonal regulation of reproductive function in men. Gonadotropin-releasing-hormone is synthesized in the hypothalamus and is transported from its site of origin via the portal blood supply to the pituitary, where it stimulates the release of both LH and FSH. LH acts on the Leydig cells to stimulate the synthesis of testosterone, and FSH acts on the Sertoli cells. For the *initiation* of spermatogenesis, these two hormones act sequentially. The high local concentrations of testosterone that bathe the seminiferous tubule facilitate the maturation of primary spermatocytes to secondary spermatocytes. Next, FSH acts to induce maturation of late spermatids to mature spermatozoa.

Testosterone and possibly FSH act on the Sertoli cell to stimulate the synthesis of the androgen-binding protein (ABP). Testosterone, bound to ABP, is transported along with mature spermatozoa to the epididymis, where the rete testis fluid is reabsorbed and testosterone is converted to dihydrotestosterone and 3α-androstanediol. In the caput epididymis, the testicular spermatozoa acquire sustained, progressive motility and fertilizing capacity. Once these maturational events have occurred, the spermatozoa are transported to the cauda epididymidis for storage. At the time of ejaculation, the epididymal spermatozoa are mixed with secretions from the prostate and seminal vesicles. Abnormalities of these important hormonal events are discussed in Chapter 2.

REFERENCES

1. Amelar, R. D.: Coagulation, liquefaction, and viscosity of human semen. J. Urol., *87*:187, 1962.
2. Amelar, R. D., and Hotchkiss, R. S.: The split ejaculate—its use in the management of male infertility. Fertil. Steril., *16*:46, 1965.
3. Baker, H. W. G. *et al.*: Testicular control of follicle-stimulating hormone secretion. Recent Progr. Horm. Res., *32*:429, 1976.
4. Batra, S. K.: Sperm transport through the vas deferens: review of hypotheses and suggestions for a quantitative model. Fertil. Steril., *25*:186, 1974.
5. Bedford, J. M.: Maturation, transport, and fate of spermatozoa in the epididymis. *In* Greep, R. O., and Astwood, E. B., Handbook of Physiology, Vol. 5, Washington, D.C. Amer. Physiol. Soc., 1975, ch. 14, pp. 303–317.
6. Blanchard, M. G., and Josso, N.: Source of the anti-Müllerian hormone synthesized by the fetal testis: Müllerian-inhibiting activity of fetal bovine Sertoli cells in tissue culture. Pediatr. Res., *8*:968, 1974.
7. Boyar, R., Finkelstein, J., Roffwarg, H., Kapen, S., Weitzman, E., and Hellman, L.: Synchronization of augmented luteinizing hormone secretion with sleep during puberty. N. Engl. J. Med., *287*:582, 1972.
8. Brendler, H.: Physiology of the prostate and seminal vesicles. *In* Campbell, M. F., and Harrison, J. H. eds., Urology. Philadelphia, W. B. Saunders Co., 1970.
9. Catt, K. J., and Dufau, M. L.: Basic concepts of the mechanism of action of peptide hormones. Biol. Reprod., *14*:1, 1976.
10. Chang, M. C., and Hunter, R. H. F.: Capacitation of mammalian sperm: biological and experimental aspects. *In* Greep, R. O., and Astwood, E. B. (eds.): Handbook of Physiology, Vol. 5. Washington, D.C., Amer. Physiol. Soc., 1975, ch. 16, pp. 339–351.
11. Christensen, A. K.: Leydig cells. *In* Greep, R. O., and Astwood, E. B. (eds.): Handbook of Physiology, Vol. 5. Washington, D.C., Amer. Physiol. Soc., 1975, ch. 3, pp. 57–94.
12. Clements, J. A., Reyes, F. I., Winter, J. S. D., and Faiman, C.: Studies on human sexual development. III. Fetal pituitary and serum, and amniotic fluid concentrations of LH, CG, and FSH. J. Clin. Endocrinol. Metab., *42*:9, 1976.
13. Clermont, Y.: Kinetics of spermatogenesis in mammals. seminiferous epithelium cycle and spermatogonial renewal. Physiol. Rev., *52*:198, 1972.
14. Clermont, Y., and Harvey, S. C.: Effect of hormones on spermatogenesis in the rat. *In* Wolstenholme, G. E. W., and O'Connor, M. (eds.): Endocrinology of the Testis. Boston, Little, Brown and Company, 1967.
15. Espiner, E. A., Veale, A. M. D., Sands, V. E., and Fitzgerald, P. H.: Familial syndrome of streak gonads and normal karyotype in five phenotypic females. N. Engl. J. Med., *283*:6, 1970.

16. Euler, U. S. V.: On the specific vasodilating and smooth muscle stimulating substance from accessory genital glands in man and certain animals (prostaglandin and vesiglandin). J. Physiol., *88*:213, 1936.
17. Fawcett, D. W.: Ultrastructure and function of the Sertoli cell. *In* Greep, R. O., and Astwood, E. B. (eds.): Handbook of Physiology, Sec. 7, Vol. 5. Washington, D.C., Amer. Physiol. Soc., 1975, ch. 2, pp. 21–55.
18. Girgis, S. M., Etriby, A., El-Hegnawy, H., and Kahil, S.: Aspermia: a survey of 49 cases. Fertil. Steril., *19*:580, 1968.
19. Greene, L. F., Kelalis, P. P., and Weeks, R. E.: Retrograde ejaculation of semen due to diabetic neuropathy: report of 4 cases. Fertil. Steril., *14*:617, 1963.
20. Gunn, S. A., and Gould, T. C.: Vasculature of the testes and adnexa. *In* Greep, R. O., and Astwood, E. B. (eds.): Handbook of Physiology, Sec. 7, Vol. 5. Washington, D.C., Amer. Physiol. Soc., 1975, ch. 5, pp. 117–142.
21. Hansson, V., Ritzén, E. M., French, F. S., and Nayfeh, S. N.: Androgen transport and receptor mechanisms in testis and epididymis. *In* Greep, R. O., and Astwood, E. B. (eds.): Handbook of Physiology, Sec. 7, Vol. 5. Washington, D.C., Amer. Physiol. Soc., 1975, ch. 7, pp. 173–201.
22. Harrison, R. G., and Winer, J. S.: Abdomino-testicular temperature gradients. J. Physiol. *107*:48, 1948.
23. Harrison, R. G., and Weiner, J. S.: The distribution of the vasal and cremasteric arteries to the testis and their functional importance. J. Anat., *83*:267, 1949.
24. Harrison, R. G., and Weiner, J. S.: Vascular patterns of the mammalian testis and their functional significance. J. Exp. Biol., *26*:304, 1949.
25. Hartman, C. G.: Science and the Safe Period. Baltimore, The Williams & Wilkins Company, 1962.
26. Heller, C. G., and Clermont, Y.: Kinetics of the germinal epithelium in man. Recent. Progr. Horm Res., *20*:545, 1964.
27. Howard, R. P., Sniffren, R. C., Simmons, F. A., and Albright, F.: Testicular deficiency: clinical and pathologic study. J. Clin. Endocrinol. Metab., *10*:121, 1950.
28. Hulka, J. F., and Davis, J. E.: Vasectomy and reversible vasocclusion. Fertil. Steril., *23*:683, 1972.
29. Johnsen, S. G.: Studies of the testicular-hypophyseal feedback mechanism in man. Acta Endocrinol. Suppl., *90*:99, 1964.
30. Jost, A.: Problems of fetal endocrinology: the gonadal and hypophyseal hormones. Recent Progr. Horm. Res., *8*:379, 1953.
31. Jost, A., Vigier, B., Prepin, J., and Perchellet, J. P.: Studies on sex differentiation in mammals. Recent. Progr. Horm. Res., *29*:1, 1973.
32. Judd, H. L., Parker, D. C., Siler, T. M., and Yen, S. S. C.: The nocturnal rise of plasma testosterone in pubertal boys. J. Clin. Endocrinol. Metab., *38*:710, 1974.
33. Kaplan, S. L., Grumbach, M. M., and Aubert, M. L.: The ontogenesis of pituitary hormones and hypothalamic factors in the human fetus: maturation of central nervous system regulation of anterior pituitary function. Recent Progr. Horm. Res., *32*:161, 1976.
34. Kedia, K. R., Markland, C., and Fraley, E. E.: Sexual function following high retroperitoneal lymphadenectomy. J. Urol., *114*:237, 1975.
35. Keiserman, W. M., Dubin, L., and Amelar, R. D.: A new type of retrograde ejaculation: report of three cases. Fertil. Steril., *25*:1071, 1974.
36. Kom, C., Mulholland, S. G., and Edson, M.: Etiology of infertility after retroperitoneal lymphadenectomy. J. Urol., *105*:528, 1971.
37. Kurzrok, R., and Lieb, C. C.: Biochemical studies of human semen: II. The action of semen on the human uterus. Proc. Soc. Exp. Biol. Med., *28*:268, 1930.
38. Lacy, D.: The seminiferous tubule in mammals. Endeavour, *26*:101, 1967.
39. Lee, P. A., Jaffe, R. B., Midgley, A. R., Jr., Kohen, F., and Niswender, G. D.: Regulation of human gonadotropins. VIII. Suppression of serum LH and FSH in adult males following exogenous testosterone administration. J. Clin. Endocrinol., *35*:636, 1973.
40. Leiter, E., and Brendler, H.: Loss of ejaculation following bilateral retroperitoneal lymphadenectomy. J. Urol., *98*:375, 1967.
41. Lipsett, M. B.: Steroid secretion by the testis in man. *In* James, V. H. T., Serio, M., and Martini, L. (eds.): The Endocrine Function of the Human Testis, Vol. 2., New York, Academic Press, 1974.

42. Lubicz-Nawrocki, C. M.: The effect of metabolites of testosterone on the viability of hamster epididymal spermatozoa. J. Endocrinol., 58:193, 1973.

43. MacLeod, J.: The effects of urinary gonadotropins following hypophysectomy and hypogonadotropic eunuchoidism. In Rosemberg, E., and Paulsen, C. A., (eds.): The Human Testis. New York, Plenum Press, 1970, pp. 577–586.

44. Mann, T.: Biochemistry of the prostate gland and its secretion. (Discussion) In Nat. Cancer Inst. Monogr., 12:235, 1963.

45. Mann, T.: Effects of pharmacological aspects on male sexual functions. J. Reprod. Fertil. (Suppl.), 4:101, 1968.

46. Mann, T.: Advances in male reproductive physiology. Fertil. Steril., 23:699, 1972.

47. Mann, T.: Biochemistry of semen. In Greep, R. O., and Astwood, E. B. (eds.): Handbook of Physiology. Sec. 7, Vol. 5. Washington D.C., Amer. Physiol. Soc., 1975, ch. 23, pp. 461–469.

48. Marshall, W. A., and Tanner, J. M.: Variations in the pattern of pubertal changes in boys. Arch. Dis. Child., 45:13, 1970.

49. McCullagh, D. R.: Dual endocrine activity of testis. Science, 76:19, 1932.

50. Means, A. R.: Biochemical effects of follicle-stimulating hormone on the testis. In Greep. R. O., and Astwood, E. B. (eds.): Handbook of Physiology, Sec. 7, Vol. 5. Washington D.C., Amer. Physiol. Soc., 1975, ch. 8, pp. 203–218.

51. Mecklenburg, R. S., Hetzel, W. D., Gulyas, B. J., and Lipsett, M. B.: Regulation of FSH secretion: use of hydroxyurea to deplete germinal epithelium. Endocrinology, 96:564, 1975.

52. Mitsuya, H., Asar, J., Sayama, K., et al.: Application of x-ray cinematography in urology. I. Mechanism of ejaculation. J. Urol., 83:86, 1960.

53. Naftolin, F., Judd, H. L., and Yen, S. S. C.: Pulsatile patterns of gonadotropins and testosterone in man: the effects of clomiphene with and without testosterone. J. Clin. Endocrinol., 36:285, 1973.

54. Ohno, S., Christian, L. C., Wachtel, S. S., and Koo, S. C.: Hormone-like role of H-Y antigen in bovine freemartin gonad. Nature, 261:597, 1976.

55. Orgebin-Crist, M. C.: Studies on the function of the epididymis. Biol. Reprod. (Suppl.), 1:155, 1969.

56. Oregin-Crist, M. C., Danzo, B. J., and Davies, J.: Endocrine control of the development and maintenance of sperm fertilizing ability in the epididymis. In Greep, R. O., and Astwood, E. B. (eds.): Handbook of Physiology, Sec. 7, Vol. 5. Washington D.C., Amer. Physiol. Soc., 1975, ch. 15, pp. 319–338.

57. Potts, I. F.: The mechanism of ejaculation. Med. J. Aust., 1:495, 1957.

58. Rieser, C.: The etiology of retrograde ejaculation and a method for insemination. Fertil. Steril., 12:488, 1961.

59. Rose, S. S.: An investigation into sterility after lumbar ganglionectomy. Brit. Med. J., 1:247, 1953.

60. Rowley, M., Teshima, J. F., and Heller, C. C.: Duration of transit of spermatozoa through the human male ductular system. Fertil. Steril., 21:390, 1970.

60a. Santen, R. J.: Is aromatization of testosterone to estradiol required for inhibition of luteinizing hormone secretion in men? J. Clin. Invest., 56:1555, 1975.

61. Schally, A. V., Mair, R. M. G., Arimura, A., and Redding, T. W.: Isolation of the luteinizing hormone and follicle-stimulating-hormone-releasing hormone from porcine hypothalami. J. Biol. Chem., 246:7230, 1971.

62. Schirger, A., and Gifford, R. W., Jr.: Guanethidine: a new antihypertensive agent; experience in the treatment of 36 patients with severe hypertension. Proc. Staff Meet. Mayo Clin., 37:100, 1962.

63. Sherins, R. J.: Clinical aspects of treatment of male infertility with gonadotropins: testicular response of some men given HCG with or without pergonal. In Mancini, R. E., and Martini, L. (eds.): Proceedings of the Serono Symposia on Male Fertility and Sterility, Vol. 5. New York, Academic Press, 1974, pp. 545–565.

64. Sherins, R. J., and Loriaux, D. L.: Studies on the role of sex steroids in the feedback control of FSH concentration in men. J. Clin. Endocrinol., 36:886, 1973.

65. Siiteri, P. K., and Wilson, J. D.: Testosterone formation and metabolism during male sexual differentiation in the human embryo. J. Clin. Endocrinol. Metab., 38:113, 1974.

66. Simpson, M. E., and Evans, H. M.: Comparison of the gametogenic and androgenic properties of testosterone propionate with those of pituitary ICSH in hypohysectomized 40-day-old male rats. Endocrinology, 39:281, 1946.

67. Sobrero, A. J., and MacLeod, J.: Immediate post-coital test. Fertil. Steril., *13*:184, 1962.
68. Spira, R.: Artificial insemination after intrathiecal injection neostigmine in a paraplegic. Lancet, *1*:670, 1960.
69. Steinberger, E.: Hormonal control of spermatogenesis. Physiol. Rev., *51*:1, 1971.
70. Swerdloff, R. S., Grover, P. K., Jacobs, H. S., and Bain, J.: Search for a substance which selectively inhibits FSH: effects of steroids and prostaglandins on serum FSH and LH levels. Steroids, *21*:703, 1973.
71. Swerdloff, R. S., and Walsh, P. C.: Testosterone and oestradiol suppression of LH and FSH in adult male rats: duration of castration, duration of treatment and combined treatment. Acta Endocrinol., *73*:11, 1973.
72. Tindall, D. J., and Means, A. R.: Concerning the hormonal regulation of androgen-binding protein in rat testis. Endocrinology, *99*:809, 1976.
73. Vanwelkenhuyzen, P.: La motilite du canal deferent. Acta Urol. Belg., *34*:385, 1966.
74. Ventura, W. P., Freund, M., Davis, J., and Pannute, C.: Influence of norepinephrine on the motility of the human vas deferens: a new hypothesis of sperm transport by the vas deferens. Fertil. Steril., *24*:68, 1973.
75. Wachtel, S. S. *et al.*: Serologic detection of a Y-linked gene in XX males and XX true hermaphrodites. N. Engl. J. Med., *295*:750, 1976.
76. Walsh, P. C., Madden, J. D., Harrod, M. J., Goldstein, J. L., MacDonald, P. C., and Wilson, J. D.: Familial incomplete male pseudohermaphroditism, type 2. Decreased dihydrotestosterone formation in pseudovaginal perineoscrotal hypospadias. N. Engl. J. Med., *291*:944, 1974.
77. Walsh, P. C., and Swerdloff, R. S.: Feedback control of FSH in the male: role of estrogen. Acta Endocrinol., *74*:449, 1973.
78. Wilson, J. D., and Lasnitzki, I.: Dihydrotestosterone formation in fetal tissues of the rabbit and rat. Endocrinology, *89*:659, 1971.
79. Winter, J. S. D., and Faiman, C.: Pituitary-gonadal relations in male children and adolescents. Pediatr. Res., *6*:126, 1972.
80. Winter, J. S. D., Faiman, C., Hobson, W. C., Prasad, A. V., and Reyes, F. I.: Pituitary-gonadal relations in infancy. 1. Patterns of serum gonadrotropin concentrations from birth to four years of age in man and chimpanzee. J. Clin. Endocrinol. Metab., *40*:545, 1975.
81. Winter, J. S. D., Hughes, I. A., Reyes, F. I., and Faiman, C.: Pituitary-gonadal relations in infancy: 2. Patterns of serum gonadal steroid concentrations in man from birth to two years of age. J. Clin. Endocrinol. Metab., *42*:679, 1976.

Chapter 2

ENDOCRINE AND CHROMOSOMAL FACTORS ASSOCIATED WITH INFERTILITY

Patrick C. Walsh, M.D.

In Chapter 1, the genetic, hormonal, biochemical, and anatomic factors that influence normal development and function of the male reproductive tract were discussed. With this background, specific defects can be identified that give rise to abnormal reproductive function in men. In this chapter, an attempt will be made to provide a pathophysiologic classifica-

33

tion of the various endocrine and chromosomal disorders that are associated with male infertility. The disorders have been divided into three broad groups: abnormalities of hypothalamic function, abnormalities of pituitary function, and abnormalities of testicular function (Fig. 2–1). In addition, the disorders of thyroid and adrenal function associated with male infertility will be discussed in this chapter.

An identifiable endocrine abnormality (hypothalamus, pituitary, testis, adrenal, or thyroid) is present in approximately 20 per cent of all infertile men.[14] However, that is probably a low estimation of the true incidence because it includes only those well-documented disorders in which the defect is virtually complete. It is likely that there are many other patients in whom partial endocrine abnormalities — e.g., subclinical hypothalamic-pituitary disease — may be responsible for varying degrees of oligospermia or

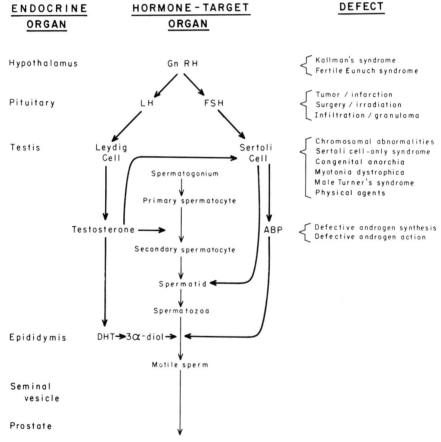

Figure 2–1. Summary of the mechanism by which various endocrinologic disorders interfere with normal reproductive function. Gonadotropin-releasing hormone (GnRH); luteinizing hormone (LH); follicle-stimulating hormone (FSH); androgen-binding protein (ABP); dihydrostestosterone (DHT); and 3α-androstaneidol (3α-diol).

abnormal sperm maturation. In addition, there are many potential sites for disorders of reproductive function, such as epididymal maturation, that are as yet unexplored. Ultimately, as the understanding of basic reproductive biology increases and as new techniques are applied to the investigation of the infertile male, the true incidence of endocrine abnormalities will be determined.

ABNORMALITIES OF HYPOTHALAMIC FUNCTION

KALLMAN'S SYNDROME

Kallman's syndrome is a familial disorder characterized by hypogonadotropic hypogonadism, anosmia, and absence of gonadotropin-releasing hormone (GnRH) secretion. This disorder is the most common form of hypogonadism aside from Klinefelter's syndrome and adult seminiferous tubular failure.[42] Because the absence of GnRH results in the failure of both LH and FSH secretion, the presenting complaint in these patients is delayed puberty rather than infertility. In boys, puberty normally begins before the age of 15, and even in patients with delayed puberty, sexual maturation is usually achieved by age 20. However, spontaneous puberty never occurs in these patients. When they are first seen they are usually tall with eunuchoidal body proportions, delayed bone age, and small, soft testes (Fig. 2–2). Kallman first described the occurrence of anosmia in this disorder in 1944. More recently, it has been recognized that in some patients the olfactory defect is partial. These patients present with hyposomia that can be recognized only by sensitive testing of olfactory function. These defects are caused by hypoplasia or aplasia of the olfactory bulbs and tracts. In addition, the patients may present with other associated somatic defects. The most common disorders associated with Kallman's syndrome are cryptorchism, cleft lip or cleft palate, and congenital deafness. More rarely, the patients may have associated color blindness, synkinesia, mental retardation, microphallus, or short fourth metacarpal. Histologically, the testes demonstrate immature seminiferous tubules containing mainly undifferentiated germinal elements with occasional early spermatogonia and absent Leydig cells. Plasma levels of LH, FSH, and testosterone are in the prepubertal range. Like prepubertal boys, there is little or no response to clomiphene stimulation.[4, 5, 51] Following treatment with HCG there is a variable response. In most patients who have never received treatment with gonadotropin, the responsiveness of serum testosterone levels to acute stimulation is impaired. However, following long-term stimulation with HCG, plasma testosterone levels usually rise into the normal range.[4, 5] In patients with bilateral cryptorchism, this response is often only minimal.[53] Although secretion of thyrotropin (TSH) and adrenocorticotropic hormone (ACTH) is normal in these disorders, occasional pa-

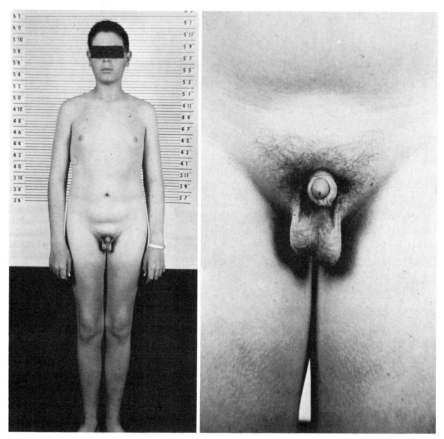

Figure 2–2. Twenty-year-old male with delayed sexual maturation, small testes and anosmia. Final diagnosis: Kallman's syndrome.

tients have deficient growth hormone secretion.[4, 5] Based on the postmortem finding of absence of the tuberal nuclei of the hypothalamus in a patient with Kallman's syndrome, de Morsier and Gauthier first suggested that the basic defect in this disorder was hypothalamic.[13] Subsequently, Naftolin and co-workers demonstrated that following the administration of GnRH to these patients, the serum gonadotropin levels were elevated.[37] More recent investigations of men with Kallman's syndrome have demonstrated that treatment with GnRH has induced full sexual maturation and the development of spermatogenesis.[36]

FERTILE EUNUCH SYNDROME

In 1950, Pasqualini and Bur described a syndrome in which spermatogenesis coexisted with the absence of Leydig cells and in which androgenic function improved after treatment with HCG.[41] Based on these findings they believed that this disorder was produced by an isolated deficiency of LH. More commonly, the term "fertile eunuch" has been used to refer to patients with eunuchoidism who have large testes, variable degrees of spermatogenesis demonstrated by testicular biopsy, and sperm counts ranging from azoospermia to the normal range.[42] Serum LH and testosterone levels are low, whereas serum FSH levels are normal. The mechanism by which spermatogenesis is maintained in these patients is not entirely clear. However, it is possible that in the presence of normal FSH levels small amounts of circulating LH are sufficient to raise the intratesticular concentration of testosterone, thereby stimulating spermatogenesis. However, the levels of LH are insufficient to raise plasma testosterone to the range necessary for normal androgenization. Santen *et al.* have reported that patients with the fertile eunuch syndrome differ from those with Kallman's syndrome only in the degree of FSH production and do not represent a separate pathogenetic entity.[51] Their conclusion is strengthened by the fact that one of their patients with the fertile eunuch syndrome also had complete anosmia. Consequently, the treatment of this disorder is similar to that of Kallman's syndrome.

OTHER HYPOTHALAMIC DISORDERS

In addition to the specific disorders in which there is isolated absence of GnRH, there are several other disorders that affect the hypothalamus and give rise to hypogonadotropism associated with a deficiency of other pituitary hormones. These conditions include neoplasms, inflammatory lesions, degenerative disorders, pituitary stalk section, and injury to the hypothalamus arising from various vascular lesions.

ABNORMALITIES OF PITUITARY FUNCTION

Pituitary insufficiency may result from nonsecretory pituitary tumors, infarction, surgical or radiation ablation, or one of a number of infiltrative or granulomatous processes.[8] If it occurs prior to puberty, growth retardation associated with adrenal or thyroid deficiency is the major clinical feature. After puberty, profound hypogonadism is one of the earliest signs. As the extent of the pituitary destruction increases, clinical evidence of other hormonal deficiencies, such as thyroid and adrenal insufficiency, presents subsequently.[8] In adult men, decreased libido, decreased potentia, and a reduction in ejaculate volume are the earliest signs of hypogonadism. The testes become small and soft, and a varying degree of damage is noted histologically. Instead of reverting to the prepubertal state, the testes show in succession maturation arrest, loss of germ cells, reduction in diameter of the tubules, and progressive thickening and hyalinization of the tunica propria.[65] In many instances the testes become completely hyalinized, and the Leydig cells progressively decrease in number and show degenerative changes. Serum LH, FSH, and testosterone levels are low. In addition, depending upon the severity of the panhypopituitarism, there may be a reduction in urinary and plasma corticosteroids, a reduction in plasma TSH associated with reduced iodine-131 thyroidal uptake, and reduced growth hormone secretion. To distinguish between hypothalamic and pituitary disorders, the thyrotropin-releasing hormone (TRH) test may be utilized in TSH-deficient patients.

There are three rare disorders affecting the hypothalamic-pituitary axis in which the precise pathophysiologic mechanism is unclear.[40] The *Prader-Labhart-Willi syndrome* is characterized by hypogonadism associated with massive obesity, mental retardation, neonatal muscle hypotonia, cryptorchism, and mild diabetes mellitus. Because the patients have uncontrollable hyperphagia and may have impaired temperature regulation, the hypogonadism appears to be of hypothalamic origin. The *Laurence-Moon-Bardet-Biedl syndrome* is a hereditary disorder characterized by retinitis pigmentosa, obesity, mental deficiency, polydactyly, and hypogonadotropic hypogonadism. Finally, in the syndrome of *familial cerebellar ataxia*, there is nerve deafness, cerebellar ataxia, and hypogonadotropic hypogonadism.

ABNORMALITIES OF TESTICULAR FUNCTION

CHROMOSOMAL ABNORMALITIES

It is well recognized that a variety of somatic chromosomal abnormalities are associated with male infertility. In a study of 1263 barren couples, Kjessler found that 6.2 per cent of the male partners had chromosomal abnormalities.[29] In those patients in whom the sperm count was less that 20 million per ml., the incidence of chromosomal abnormalities was only 1.9 per cent, but if the sperm count was less than 10 million, the incidence increased to 11 per cent. In patients with azoospermia, 21 per cent had significant chromosomal abnormalities. In the series of de Krester *et al.* 11 of 56 patients with oligospermia or azoospermia demonstrated chromosomal abnormalities.[10] More recently, Hendry *et al.* investigated 204 subfertile men.[23] In this series, 7 (3.5 per cent) demonstrated definite somatic chromosomal abnormalities, and 21 (10.5 per cent) showed variations of the Y chromosome. These studies emphasize the necessity of cytogenetic studies in patients with severe oligospermia and azoospermia. Table 2–1 lists the various sex chromosomal and autosomal defects that have been associated with male infertility.

Klinefelter's Syndrome. In 1942, Klinefelter, Reifenstein, and Albright described a disorder characterized by gynecomastia, azoospermia,

Table 2–1 CHROMOSOMAL ABNORMALITIES ASSOCIATED
WITH MALE INFERTILITY

SEX CHROMOSOMAL
XXY
XY/XXY
XXYY
XXXY
XXXXY
XYY
XX
XY/XO
XY/XX
XY q+/q−

AUTOSOMAL
D–D translocations
Ring chromosomal abnormalities
Reciprocal translocations
Robertsonian aberrations

atrophic testes, increased urinary excretion of pituitary gonadotropins, and various degrees of underandrogenization (Fig. 2–3).[30] Since that time, it has been recognized that Klinefelter's syndrome is the most common form of male hypogonadism, affecting 0.2 per cent of the male population. The fundamental defect responsible for Klinefelter's syndrome is the presence of two or more X chromosomes. Paulsen and co-workers have suggested that any phenotypic male who demonstrates two or more X chromosomes plus at least one Y chromosome in all or part of his body tissue should be included in this syndrome.[31] In the classic form of the disorder, defective spermatogenesis, azoospermia, and small, firm testes (usually less than 2.0 cm. and always less than 3.5 cm. in length) are present in virtually all patients. The typical histologic pattern of the testes in the patient with the classical form of Klinefelter's syndrome consists of hyalinization and fibrosis of the seminiferous tubules and adenomatous clumping of the Leydig cells.[42] With the exception of gynecomastia, all of the remaining abnormalities in patients with Klinefelter's syndrome are related to decreased Leydig cell function (Table 2–2). The gynecomastia usually occurs first during adolescence, is usually bilateral and painless, and may become disfiguring. Because its assessment is subjective, the incidence of 50 per cent should be regarded as a minimal figure.

In the classic form of the syndrome, plasma and urinary LH and FSH levels are high and, on the average, plasma testosterone levels are only 50 per cent of normal. However, many patients have testosterone values that fall within the normal range, particularly when the plasma LH levels are high. Because of this variability in plasma testosterone levels, serum LH levels may be a more accurate and sensitive indication of Leydig cell function.[42]

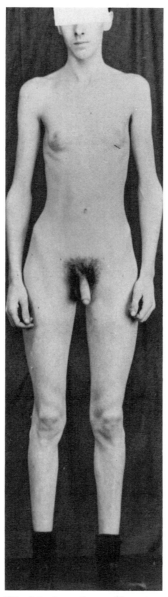

Figure 2–3.   A patient with Klinefelter's syndrome. (Courtesy of Dr. Harry F. Klinefelter.)

In addition to the classic form approximately 30 other karyotypic varieties of Klinefelter's syndrome have been described, including XY/XXXY, XXYY, XXXY, XXXXY, and a variety of mosaics. The most common of these clinical variants is the 46XY/47XXY mosaic. In this form of the disorder, the testes may be normal in size, fertility may be present in isolated cases, and the endocrine abnormalities are less severe.[38]

Table 2–2 CLINICAL FEATURES IN XXY AND XY/XXY KLINEFELTER'S SYNDROME*

	XXY (%)	XY/XXY (%)
Small testes	99	73
Azoospermia	93	50
Diminished facial hair	77	64
Gynecomastia	55	33
Small penis	41	21
Increased gonadotropins	75	33
Decreased testosterone	79	33

*From Paulsen, C. A., Gordon, D. L., Carpenter, R. W. et al.: Klinefelter's syndrome and its variants: hormonal and chromosomal study. Recent Progr. Horm. Res., 24:321, 1968.

Because in many cases the mosaicism is present in only a limited number of tissues, this variant may be difficult to diagnose (Table 2–2). However, in all patients the mosaicism is present in the testes.

XYY Syndrome. The incidence of a 47XYY karyotype is approximately the same as that of Klinefelter's syndrome, affecting about 0.2 per cent of the male population. However, the phenotypic expression of this disorder is much more variable. Some studies have suggested that these patients are especially likely to be found in correctional facilities for antisocial behavior because the incidence of this karyotype in the prison population is tenfold higher than in newborn males.[24, 61] Characteristically, these patients are tall and have had pustular acne. Spermatogenesis may be normal, minimally affected, or severely damaged. In those patients with low sperm counts, spermatogenic arrest has been a common finding. Although some studies have suggested that plasma gonadotropin and testosterone levels are normal in these individuals, investigations of large populations suggest that the findings are heterogeneous and that moderate hypogonadism is present in some individuals.[3] In others, plasma testosterone levels have been elevated. With greater experience, the true incidence of these clinical and endocrinologic abnormalities will become clearer.

The Sex-Reversal Syndrome. Since 1964, approximately 45 men with a 46XX karyotype have been reported.[12, 26] Clinically, these patients resemble patients with Klinefelter's syndrome and present with a male phenotype, small testes, gynecomastia, and azoospermia. Histologically, the adult testes demonstrate absence of spermatogenesis, hyalinization of the tubules, and Leydig cell hyperplasia. Recently, Wachtel et al. have demonstrated that in patients with this disorder the H-Y antigen is present.[57] Consequently, these data suggest that the genetic material responsible for the testis-determining factor is present in these individuals and that in truth this disorder represents one more variant of Klinefelter's syndrome, in which two X chromosomes coexist with all or part of a Y chromosome.

Sex Chromosomal Abnormalities Associated with Intersexuality. In this classification there are two disorders that may present with infertility. Although typically patients with either mixed gonadal dysgenesis or true hermaphroditism are first diagnosed at birth, these disorders in their mildest forms may not be detected until adulthood.

Mixed gonadal dysgenesis is the more common disorder; in some series it has been reported to be the second most frequent cause of ambiguous genitalia in the neonate, ranking only after adrenocortical hyperplasia. Phenotypically, these patients are incompletely virilized, and over 60 per cent have been reared as females.[9] However, in several instances normal virilization including a complete phallic urethra has been reported. All patients have a uterus, a vagina, and at least one fallopian tube; typically there is a testis on one side and a streak gonad on the other.[9] The most common karyotype is 45XO/46XY. Postpubertally, although the patients develop masculine features, the seminiferous tubules lack all germinal elements and contain only Sertoli cells. Finally, more than 25 per cent of the patients who are reared as males will develop a testicular tumor, typically a gonadoblastoma.

True hermaphroditism, a condition in which both ovarian and testicular tissue is present, is a rare disorder, and only approximately 300 cases have been reported in the literature. Unlike mixed gonadal dysgenesis, these patients are relatively well masculinized, and for this reason 60 to 75 per cent have been reared as males. The predominant internal ductal structures vary with the gonad that is present. Although the most common karyotype is 46XX, recent evidence suggests that these patients have an H-Y antigen.[57] Fertility in patients that have been reared as males has been reported only occasionally. However, with earlier recognition and surgical correction it is hoped that the prospects for fertility can be improved.

Y Chromosomal Abnormalities. Several variants of the Y chromosome have been reported to be associated with male infertility. In a recent study of 200 patients, abnormalities of the Y chromosome were present in 10.5 per cent: 13 patients were 46XYq+ and 2 were 46XYq− (depending on the addition or deletion of the long arm of the Y).[23] However, because Y chromosomal abnormalities are common and may be present in fertile individuals, it is difficult to be certain of the pathogenetic significance of their presence in infertile men.

Autosomal Abnormalities. An assortment of autosomal abnormalities has been reported to be associated with male infertility. These have included D-D translocations, ring chromosomal abnormalities, reciprocal translocations, and Robertsonian aberrations.[29] In most instances, the association of these abnormalities with infertility has been documented in only isolated cases—proof awaits a large prospective study. However, with the new chromosomal banding techniques, specific identification of each chromosome pair is possible, and consequently the various translocations can be more precisely described. These techniques have recently been used in the investigation of a family in which there was an association between a D-group chromosomal translocation and defective spermatogenesis.[45] With wilder utilization of these techniques, it may be determined that certain translocations within the D-group are associated with spermatogenic defects while others lack such an association.

SERTOLI CELL–ONLY SYNDROME

In 1947, del Castillo *et al.* described a syndrome in which azoospermia was associated with testicular tubules that were smaller than normal and were devoid of germinal epithelium.[11] In a series of 1294 consecutive cases of male infertility, this disorder was present in 3.4 per cent of the patients.[14] In this same series, the incidence of Klinefelter's syndrome was 2.7 per cent. Patients with this disorder present with azoospermia and testes that are normal in consistency but slightly smaller than normal in size. Histologically, the seminiferous tubules are moderately reduced in size and all germinal elements are absent, but there is no hyalinization or peritubular fibrosis. Morphologically, the Leydig cells are normal. Serum LH and testosterone levels are usually normal, but plasma FSH levels are increased. Although some investigators have suggested that congenital absence of germ cells is the basis for this syndrome, there is no direct evidence to support this thesis.[42]

CONGENITAL ANORCHIA

This term has been used to refer to phenotypic males who present with eunuchoidism, nonpalpable testes, and a normal 46XY karyotype, and who have complete development of the wolffian system but absence of the müllerian duct structures and gonads. More than 50 cases of this disorder have been reported.[16] Prepubertally, these patients are indistinguishable from boys with bilateral cryptorchism, and often the diagnosis is not made until the time of surgical exploration. If the patients are not evaluated until later in life, puberty will have failed to occur, since there is no gonadal tissue to respond to endogenous gonadotropin stimulation. The etiology of this disorder is unclear. Because these patients have virilization of the wolffian ducts, regression of the müllerian structures, masculinization of the urogenital sinus and external genitalia, and normal phallic development, the failure of testicular tissue must occur sometime after the first and most likely after the second trimester of pregnancy. Prepubertally, the diagnosis can be established with the aid of serum gonadotropin and HCG stimulation tests. Plasma LH and FSH levels will be elevated, and there is no response to HCG stimulation.[64]

MYOTONIA DYSTROPHICA

In this rare disorder, myotonia, progressive muscular atrophy, frontal baldness, and cataracts are associated with testicular atrophy. Hypogonadism, which develops in approximately 80 per cent of these patients with age, is characterized by seminiferous tubular failure with normal Leydig cell function.[42] The frontal baldness does not appear to be directly related to the degree of hypogonadism. The findings on testicular biopsy range from complete hyalinization and fibrosis of the seminiferous tubules to moderate derangement of spermatogenesis.[42] As a reflection of the injury to the seminiferous tubules, serum FSH levels are often elevated. This disorder is inherited as an autosomal dominant trait.

MALE TURNER'S SYNDROME (NOONAN'S SYNDROME; ULLRICH'S SYNDROME; XX OR XY TURNER'S PHENOTYPE)

This disorder, which is inherited as an autosomal dominant mutation, affects both male and female subjects with normal karyotypes and is characterized by the presence of a webbed neck, short stature, congenital heart disease, cubitus valgus, and other congenital defects. This disorder should not be confused with mixed gonadal dysgenesis, in which patients with XO/XY mosaicism may have some of the somatic anomalies typical of Turner's syndrome.[9] In the typical patient with male Turner's syndrome, the most common cardiac malformations have been pulmonic stenosis and atrial septal defects. In males with this disorder, cryptorchism is common, and the testes are often hypoplastic and exhibit germinal aplasia. Plasma testosterone levels may be low, and serum LH and FSH levels may be elevated postpubertally. However, some affected individuals have descended testes and normal testicular function and are fertile.

PHYSICAL AGENTS

As discussed later, a variety of physical agents may induce damage to the seminiferous tubules. Increased temperature secondary to an acute febrile illness or cryptorchism, irradiation, and various drugs are the most common causes of such damage. In these patients, although serum LH and testosterone levels are normal, elevated levels of plasma FSH are present. A detailed discussion of these disorders is presented in Chapter 4.

DEFECTIVE ANDROGEN SYNTHESIS

For spermatogenesis to progress beyond the stage of the pachytene spermatocyte, testosterone must be present in high concentrations within the seminiferous tubules. Consequently, any disorder that leads to a defect in testosterone synthesis will markedly inhibit spermatogenesis. There are a variety of hereditary disorders in which defective testosterone synthesis is associated with inadequate virilization during embryogenesis, thereby producing ambiguous genitalia in the male. In addition, several acquired disorders in adult men may give rise to deficient synthesis of testosterone and abnormal spermatogenesis.

There are five enzymatic steps necessary for the conversion of cholesterol to testosterone (Fig. 2–4). A defect in any one of these enzymes may give rise to inadequate testosterone synthesis *in utero,* resulting in incomplete virilization and ambiguous genitalia in male infants. Three of these enzymes (20,22-desmolase,[28] 3β-hydroxysteroid dehydrogenase,[55] and 17-hydroxylase[39]) are common to the synthesis of adrenal hormones as well as androgens; consequently, a deficiency of one of these enzymes results in congenital adrenal hyperplasia as well as ambiguous genitalia in male infants. The other two enzymes (17,20-desmolase[66] and 17β-hydroxy-

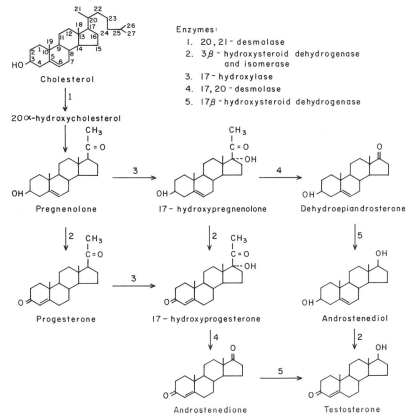

Figure 2–4. Metabolic pathway for the conversion of cholesterol to testosterone in the testes.

steroid dehydrogenase[17]) are unique to the pathway of androgen synthesis, and therefore their deficiency results only in inadequate virilization and not in congenital adrenal hyperplasia. The phenotypic expression of these disorders is variable owing to the varying severity of the enzymatic defect. Consequently, the spectrum of clinical presentation varies from patients with only mild hypospadias to those with female external genitalia and intra-abdominal testes. All patients have regression of the müllerian ducts, but virilization of the wolffian ducts, urogenital sinus, and urogenital tubercle varies. At puberty, the degree of sexual maturation varies from florid virilization with or without gynecomastia to complete failure. Virtually every patient reported up to the present time has had some abnormality of the external genitalia. However, it is possible that patients with these enzymatic defects in their mildest form could present with infertility as the only manifestation. The diagnosis is based on the demonstration of inadequate testosterone synthesis and elevated gonadotropin secretion. However, in patients with incomplete defects, there may be adequate compensation so that the steady state of concentration of testosterone may be within the normal statistical range. In these instances, the diagnosis can be made only by measuring the steroids that accumulate proximal to the metabolic block in question. The pattern of inheritance of these disorders is variable. Based on the available evidence, the 17-hydroxylase and 3β-hydroxysteroid dehydrogenase deficiencies are inherited as autosomal recessive traits, and the 17,20-desmolase and 17β-hydroxysteroid dehydrogenase deficiencies are inherited either as autosomal recessive or X-linked recessive traits. Insufficient data are available to warrant any conclusions about the inheritance of the 20,22-desmolase defect. At the present time, fertility has not been reported in any patient with these abnormalities.

    In addition to the congenital disorders that give rise to defective androgen synthesis, infertility in adult men may be induced by acquired defects in the synthesis of testosterone produced by treatment with drugs, renal failure, or alcoholic cirrhosis. There are several drugs that block one or more of the enzymes necessary for the synthesis of testosterone. Aminoglutethimide inhibits the side chain cleavage of cholesterol and subsequent hydroxylation; spironolactone and cyproterone acetate act further down the pathway at the 17,20-desmolase enzyme; and cyanoketone, 17β-estradiol, hydroxymethylene, and medrogestone inhibit the 3β-hydroxysteroid dehydrogenase enzyme.[58] More commonly, testosterone therapy may induce infertility by indirectly suppressing testosterone synthesis. It is known that when testosterone is administered to normal men, testicular atrophy and azoospermia result. Because total urinary gonadotropins are suppressed and Leydig cell atrophy occurs, it was assumed that inhibition of LH and FSH produced this suppression of spermatogenesis.[22] However, Heller *et al.* were the first to note that the azoospermia that resulted from testosterone therapy could be reversed by simultaneous treatment with HCG (which has LH-like activity).[21] They suggested that testosterone therapy inhibits spermatogenesis by producing an isolated suppression of LH levels, thereby lowering androgen production by the Leydig cells. Consequently, although testosterone therapy may maintain plasma testosterone at normal levels, there is a reduction in the concentration of testosterone within the testes because the Leydig cell synthesis of testosterone is suppressed, and spermatogenesis is thereby suppressed. It is apparent that FSH inhibition is not required for testosterone to suppress spermatogenesis.[60]

The mechanism responsible for infertility in patients with renal failure is not completely understood. However, there is data suggesting that defective testosterone synthesis may play a role. In men, uremia is associated with loss of libido, reduced potentia, sterility, testicular atrophy, and gynecomastia. Commonly, testicular biopsies demonstrate spermatogenic arrest with no maturation beyond the primary spermatocyte level.[44] Leydig cell morphology is normal, and there is no thickening of the basement membrane. Although the precise nature of the dysfunction in the hypothalamic-pituitary-gonadal axis in these patients has not been ascertained, and it is possible that more than one defect may exist, most authors have found reduced levels of plasma testosterone in affected patients. Stewart-Bentley et al. reported that plasma testosterone levels in uremic men were subnormal and that the blood production rate of testosterone was markedly decreased.[56] However, following dialysis plasma testosterone levels increased to the normal range, and testosterone production more than doubled. In these patients, the serum LH levels were elevated, and it was therefore concluded that the decreased testosterone production was due to Leydig cell dysfunction. In support of these findings is the fact that uremic men usually have a normal LH surge following treatment with clomiphene or GnRH.[54, 56] However, because they fail to hypersecrete gonadotropin in response to GnRH the possibility of a hypothalamic-pituitary deficiency cannot be excluded.[54]

The precise etiology of hypogonadism and gynecomastia in patients with alcoholic cirrhosis is unclear. In detailed endocrinologic studies, men with this disorder have been noted to have decreased plasma testosterone levels and decreased metabolic clearance rates, increased binding of testosterone to plasma proteins, increased plasma estradiol and enhanced production rates of estradiol, and low, normal, or moderately elevated serum gonadotropin levels.[18] On the basis of these findings, it is likely that combined hypothalamic-pituitary and testicular dysfunction is responsible for this disorder. Recent studies have suggested that when normal volunteers are subjected to the subacute administration of moderate amounts of alcohol (250 ml. per day) plasma testosterone and testosterone production rates fall.[18] Because this occurs in some patients without suppression of serum LH levels, a direct effect on the Leydig cell is likely. However, with chronic administration of alcohol, gonadotropin levels are suppressed and testosterone clearance increases secondary to enhanced hepatic testosterone A-ring reductase activity. Consequently, in the absence of hepatic failure, excessive alcohol consumption can lower plasma testosterone levels by directly suppressing Leydig cell synthesis, by increasing testosterone metabolic clearance rates, and by suppressing gonadotropins.

DEFECTIVE ANDROGEN ACTION

Although it has been known for many years that the growth and function of the secondary organs of reproduction are under the regulation of androgen, only relatively recently has the mechanism responsible for the action of androgen been well defined. It is widely accepted that steroidal hormones promote the synthesis of ribonucleic acid and proteins by acting within the nucleus of various target tissues. In 1968, Bruchovsky and Wilson[6] and Anderson and Liao demonstrated that, following the administration of testosterone to rats, 5α-dihydrotestosterone was the major metabolite isolated from the nuclei of the ventral prostate. This observation strongly suggests that dihydrotestosterone was the major intracellular metabolite responsible for the action of androgen in the prostate (Fig. 1–1). Once testosterone is converted to dihydrotestosterone, dihydrotestosterone binds to a high affinity macromolecular protein, the receptor, which is initially located in the cytoplasm. Next, this steroid-receptor complex undergoes a temperature-dependent physical change that enables the complex to translocate to the nucleus and bind to acceptor substances located on the chromatin. It is assumed that these events then activate transcription and result in the formation of messenger RNA and increased protein synthesis (Fig. 2–5). Based on these principles, a defect in one or more of the mechanisms that mediates the action of androgen on the target organ may

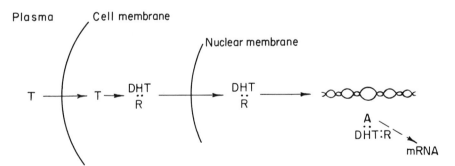

Figure 2–5. Proposed mechanism by which androgens stimulate protein synthesis within target tissues. Testosterone (T) crosses the plasma membrane by simple diffusion and is converted to dihydrotestosterone (DHT). DHT combines with the cytoplasmic receptor (R) to form the dihydrotestosterone-receptor complex. This complex is transferred to the nucleus where it combines with acceptors (A) located on the chromatin. These events stimulate the synthesis of messenger RNA (mRNA) and then protein synthesis.

lead to abnormal spermatogenesis. Because these disorders also affect virilization *in utero,* patients with a defect in androgen action present clinically with infertility associated with ambiguous genitalia.

Based on endocrinologic, biochemical, and genetic studies, four distinct forms of defective androgen action can be identified: (1) complete testicular feminization; (2) incomplete testicular feminization; (3) familial incomplete male pseudohermaphroditism, type 1; and (4) familial incomplete male pseudohermaphroditism, type 2. A detailed discussion of only one of these disorders (incomplete male pseudohermaphroditism, type 1) will be provided here because patients with the other disorders are usually reared as females. In complete testicular feminization, 46XY patients with bilateral testes that are capable of normal testosterone synthesis differentiate as phenotypic females.[63] At puberty feminization occurs but there is absence of axillary and pubic hair. This disorder, which is inherited as an X-linked recessive trait, represents the most complete form of androgen resistance that occurs in man. The primary defect in this disorder appears to be an inherited abnormality in the amount or function of the androgen receptor.[27] Patients with incomplete testicular feminization also have a 46XY karyotype, bilateral testes, and normal testosterone synthesis.[34] Clinically, these patients are slightly more virilized than subjects with the testicular feminization syndrome, and in most cases the family history is uninformative. Recent studies suggest that in this disorder there is a partial defect in the androgen receptor.[19] Finally, most patients with incomplete male pseudohermaphroditism, type 2, a disorder that is also termed pseudovaginal perineoscrotal hypospadias, have been reared as females.[59] The distinctive characteristics of this disorder are the presence of normal wolffian duct structures, severe perineoscrotal hypospadias with a hooded prepuce, masculinization to a variable degree at the time of puberty, and an autosomal recessive inheritance. Recent studies have demonstrated that deficient dihydrotestosterone formation is the fundamental defect in this disorder.[59]

The term familial incomplete male pseudohermaphroditism, type 1, has been used to identify a group of disorders in which the most common presentation is that of a male with hypospadias, azoospermia, incomplete virilization at the time of puberty, gynecomastia, and an X-linked inheritance.[62] Actually, this term refers to a complete spectrum of clinical disorders ranging from patients with almost complete absence of virilization to the mildest form in which patients present with infertility and gynecomastia. Originally, at least four separate clinical disorders were described that fit into this broad category: (1) Lubs syndrome, a disorder in which phenotypic females have partial wolffian duct development, partial labioscrotal fusion, normal pubic and axillary hair, and a masculine skeletal development;[33] (2) Gilbert-Dreyfus syndrome, in which phenotypic males present with a small phallus, hypospadias, incomplete wolffian duct structures, and gynecomastia;[15] (3) Reifenstein's syndrome, in which phenotypic males present with perineal hypospadias, a bifid scrotum, and gynecomastia at puberty;[49] (4) Rosewater's syndrome, the mildest form, in which males present with gynecomastia and infertility.[50] However, based on the analysis of several large pedigrees, it has been determined that individual affected members of the same family may exhibit phenotypes that correspond to either the most mild (Rosewater's syndrome) or the most severe (Lubs syndrome) defects described above.[62] Consequently, because the inheritance in these disorders appears to be X-linked, Wilson and co-workers concluded that these disorders most likely represent variable manifestations of a single gene mutation; they proposed the term familial incomplete male pseudohermaphoditism, type 1, to identify this group.[62]

Typically, the patients present with perineal hypospadias, atrophic testes, incomplete virilization at puberty, and gynecomastia (Fig. 2–6). At puberty, pubic and axillary hair develop, but chest and facial hair is sparse. In the less severely affected individuals, the principal manifestations are sterility, a bifid scrotum, incomplete virilization at puberty, and gynecomastia. Cryptorchism is common, and the testes remain small in size. Histologically, the testes demonstrate normal Leydig cells and tubules that contain both germinal cells and Sertoli cells, although there is usually no maturation beyond the primary spermatocyte. Plasma testosterone and LH levels are high, suggesting that androgen resistance is present and that there is a defect in the feedback control of testosterone on the hypothalamus.[62] Treatment with testosterone in large doses fails both to suppress plasma LH to normal and to induce further sexual maturation. Recent studies have suggested that in patients with this disorder, the levels of cytoplasmic receptor proteins are low.[19]

ABNORMALITIES OF THYROID FUNCTION

Thyroid dysfunction is a rare cause of male infertility. Dubin and Amelar reported that of 1294 consecutive male patients with infertility thyroid disease was the causative factor in only 0.6 per cent.[14] Because the infertility associated with thyroid disorders may be reversible with proper medical management, this possibility should be considered in evaluating patients. However, the rare occurrence of this disorder strongly weighs against the empirical use of thyroid hormones for the treatment of idiopathic oligospermia.

Adult men with hypothyroidism may present with vague nonspecific symptoms such as lethargy, constipation, sensitivity to cold, and loss of libido. With progression of the disease, the patients become apathetic and listless, and develop loss of hair, dry skin, periorbital puffiness, and occasionally deafness.[25] Eventually, fullblown myxedema occurs, resulting in an enlarged tongue, hoarseness, nonpitting edema, and extreme mental and physical lethargy. In patients with hypothyroidism, serum thyroxine and

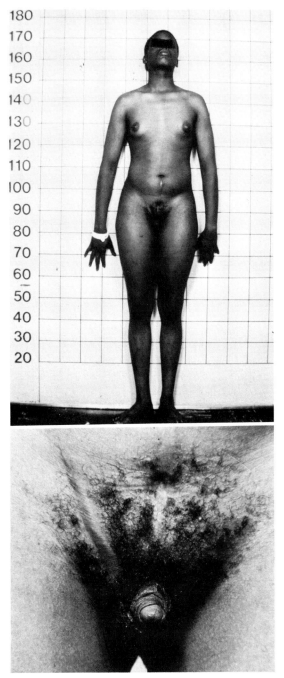

Figure 2-6. Sixteen-year-old boy with microphallus, surgically corrected hypospadias, gynecomastia, and azoospermia typical of the phenotype in familial incomplete male pseudo-hermaphroditism, type 1.

tri-iodothyronine levels are low, thyroid-binding globulin is normal or high, and free thyroxine is low.

Hyperthyroidism has occasionally caused infertility. However, because hyperthyroid patients rarely consult a physician for the primary complaint of infertility, attention is usually focused on other manifestations of the disease, and the fertility status of the patient is often not evaluated. Consequently, the true incidence and etiology of impaired infertility in this disorder are not well understood. Recently, Clyde *et al.* studied three young men with marked hyperthyroidism and secondary infertility.[7] These patients had increased serum thyroxine and tri-iodothyronine levels and increased iodine-131 uptake. In addition, the serum levels of testosterone and LH were elevated, and in each case these values returned to normal when euthyroidism was attained. Because maturation arrest at the primary spermatocyte level was found on testicular biopsy in one patient, it is tempting to speculate that some abnormality of androgen metabolism is responsible for the defective spermatogenesis in this disorder. However, the suppression of spermatogenesis in these patients may be the consequence of nonspecific factors such as stress or increased temperature.

ABNORMALITIES OF ADRENAL FUNCTION

Well-documented cases of adrenal dysfunction giving rise to male infertility are rare. In patients with Addison's disease, impotence and decreased libido are relatively common. However, Paulsen states that the impaired testicular function in this disorder is most likely caused by a nonspecific reduction in pituitary function.[42] Even in patients with normal gonadotropin secretion and testicular function, the impairment of potentia and libido is probably secondary to the weakness that occurs with adrenal insufficiency.

Congenital adrenal hyperplasia is the one disorder of adrenal function that is clearly responsible for abnormal spermatogenesis. In males with the most common forms of the disorder, a deficiency of 21-hydroxylase or 11-hydroxylase, the disease is usually not recognized at birth unless overt adrenal insufficiency develops. However, there is early growth and maturation of the genitalia and early appearance of secondary sexual characteristics. Acne, coarsening of the voice, frequent erections, and excessive muscular development are noticeable within the first few years of life. The testes usually remain infantile in size despite the acceleration of masculinization. If the patients are reared to adulthood without treatment with cortisone, most of them are clinically unremarkable except for small stature, small testes, and sterility. The hypogonadism in these patients is produced by suppression of gonadotropins by androgen of adrenal origin.[35, 46] Treatment with cortisone suppresses production of adrenal androgen and restores the pulsatile release of LH.[48] Sustained suppression of adrenal androgens results in restoration of fertility.

Some authors have suggested that a mild form of congenital adrenal hyperplasia, possibly acquired, may play a significant role in the pathogenesis of male infertility. In this proposed form of the disorder, there is no history of precocious puberty and no alterations in the physical appearance of the patients. The semen demonstrates a "stress pattern" with oligospermia, poor sperm motility, and an increase in immature forms in the ejaculate.[1] The diagnosis has been based on the finding of elevated 17-ketosteroid levels in the urine. However, since elevations of 17-ketosteroids may be nonspecific, better documentation is necessary before one can make this diagnosis with confidence. In the 21-hydroxylase deficiency, elevated serum levels of 17-hydroxyprogesterone and increased urinary pregnanetriol should be present. In the 11-hydroxylase deficiency, there should be elevated serum levels of 11-deoxycortisol and increased urinary excretion of tetrahydro S. Unless these abnormalities can be demonstrated, the empirical use of cortisone suppression in patients with idiopathic oligospermia should be discouraged.

REFERENCES

1. Amelar, R. D., and Dubin, L.: Male infertility. Current diagnosis and treatment. Urology, *1*:1, 1973.
2. Anderson, K. M., and Liao, S.: Selective retention of dihydrotestosterone by prostatic nuclei. Nature, *219*:277, 1968.
3. Baghdassarian, A., Bayard, F., Borgaonkar, D. S., Arnold, E. A., Solez, K., and Migeon, C. D.: Testicular function in XYY men. Johns Hopkins Med. J., *136*:15, 1975.
4. Bardin, C. W., Ross, G. T., Rifkind, A. B., Cargille, C. M., and Lipsett, M. B.: Studies of the pituitary-Leydig cell axis in young men with hypogonadotropic hypogonadism and hyposmia: comparison with normal men, prepubertal boys, and hypopituitary patients. J. Clin. Invest., *48*:2046, 1969.
5. Boyar, R. M., Finkelstein, J. W., Witkin, M., Kapen, S., Weitzmann, E., and Hellman, L.: Studies of endocrine function in isolated gonadotropin deficiency. J. Clin. Endocrinol. Metab., *36*:64, 1973.
6. Bruchovsky, N., and Wilson, J. D.: The conversion of testosterone to 5α-androstan-17β-ol-3-one by rat prostate in vivo and in vitro. J. Biol. Chem., *243*:2012, 1968.
7. Clyde, H. R., Walsh, P. C., and English, R. W.: Elevated plasma testosterone and gonadotropin levels in infertile males with hyperthyroidism. Fertil. Steril., *27*:662, 1976.
8. Daughaday, W. H.: The adenohypophysis. *In* Williams, R. H. (ed.): Textbook of Endocrinology, 5th ed. Philadelphia, W. B. Saunders Co., 1974, p. 31–79.
9. Davidoff, F., and Federman, D. D.: Mixed gonadal dysgenesis. Pediatrics, *52*:725–747, 1973.
10. deKrester, D. M., Burger, H. G., Fortune, D., Hudson, B., Long, A. R., Paulsen, C. A., and Taft, H. P.: Hormonal, histological, and chromosomal studies. J. Clin. Endocrinol. Metab., *35*:392, 1972.
11. del Castillo, E., Trabucco, A., and de La Balze, F.: Syndrome produced by absence of germinal epithelium without impairment of the Sertoli cells. J. Clin. Endocrinol. Metab., *7*:493, 1947.
12. De la Chapelle, A.: Nature and origin of males with XX sex chromosomes. Amer. J. Hum. Genet., *24*:71–105, 1972.
13. De Morsier, G., and Gauthier, G.: La dysplasia olfacto-genitale. Pathol. Biol. (Paris), *11*:1267, 1963.
14. Dubin, L., and Amelar, R. D.: Etiologic factors in 1294 consecutive cases of male infertility. Fertil. Steril., *22*:469, 1971.

15. Gilbert-Dreyfus, S., Sebaoun, C. I. A., and Belaisch, J.: Etude d'un cas familial d'androgynoidisine avec hypospadias grave, gynecomastie et hyperoestrogenie. Ann. Endocrinol. (Paris), *18*:93, 1957.

16. Glenn, J. F., and McPherson, H. T.: Anorchism: definition of a clinical entity. J. Urol., *105*:265, 1971.

17. Goebelsman, U., Horton, R., Mestman, J. H., Arce, J. J., Nagata, Y., Nakamura, R. M., Thorneycroft, I. H., and Mishell, D. R., Jr.: Male pseudohermaphroditism due to testicular 17β-hydroxysteroid dehydrogenase deficiency. J. Clin. Endocrinol. Metab., *36*:867, 1973.

18. Gordon, G. G., Altman, K., Southern, A. L., Rubin, E., and Lieber, C. S.: Effect of alcohol (ethanol) administration on sex-hormone metabolism in normal men. N. Engl. J. Med., *295*:793, 1976.

19. Griffin, J. E., Punyashthiti, K., and Loilson, J. D.: Dihydrotestosterone binding by cultured human fibroblasts. Comparison of cells from control subjects and from patients with hereditary male pseudohermaphroditism due to androgen resistance. J. Clin. Invest., *57*:1342, 1976.

20. Hall, B. D., and Smith, D. W.: Prader-Willi syndrome. A resume of 32 cases including an instance of affected first cousins, one of whom is of normal stature and intelligence. J. Pediatr., *81*:286, 1972.

21. Heller, C. G., Morse, H. C., Su, U., and Rowley, M. J.: The role of FSH, ICSH, and endogenous testosterone during testicular suppression by exogenous testosterone in normal men. *In* Rosemberg, E., and Paulsen, C. A. (eds.): The Human Testis. New York, Plenum Press, 1970, pp. 240–257.

22. Heller, C. G., Nelson, W. O., Hill, I. B., Henderson, E., Maddock, W. O., Jungck, E. C., Paulsen, C. A., and Mortimore, G. E.: Improvement in spermatogenesis following depression of the human testis with testosterone. Fertil. Steril., *1*:415, 1950.

23. Hendry, W. F., Polani, P. E., Pugh, R. C. B., Sommerville, I. F., and Wallace, D. M.: 200 infertile males: correlation of chromosome, histological, endocrine, and clinical studies. Brit. J. Urol., *47*:899, 1976.

24. Hook, E. B.: Behavioral implication of the human XYY genotype. Science, *179*:139, 1973.

25. Ingbar, S. H., and Woeber, K. A.: The thyroid gland. *In* Williams, R. H. (ed.): Textbook of Endocrinology, 5th ed. Philadelphia, W. B. Saunders Co., 1974, p. 95–232.

26. Kasdan, R., Nankin, H. R., Troen, P., Wald, N., Pan, S., and Yanaihara, T.: Paternal transmission of maleness of XX human beings. N. Engl. J. Med., *288*:539, 1973.

27. Keenan, B. S., Meyer, W. J., III, Hadjian, A. J., Jones, H. W., and Migeon, C. J.: Syndrome of androgen insensitivity in man: absence of 5α-dihydrotestosterone binding protein in skin fibroblasts. J. Clin. Endocrinol. Metab., *38*:1143, 1974.

28. Kirkland, R. T., Kirkland, J. L., Johnson, C. M., Horning, M. G., Librik, L., and Clayton, G. W.: Congenital lipoid adrenal hyperplasia in an 8-year old phenotypic female. J. Clin. Endocrinol. Metab., *36*:488, 1973.

29. Kjessler, B.: Fracteurs génétiques dans la subfertilé male humaine. *In* Fécondité et Stérilité du Male. Acquisitions recéntes. Paris, Masson et Cie, 1972.

30. Klinefelter, H. F., Jr., Reifenstein, E. C., Jr., and Albright, F.: Syndrome characterized by gynecomastia, aspermatogenesis, without A-Leydigism, and increased excretion of follicle-stimulating hormone. J. Clin. Endocrinol. Metabl., *2*:615, 1942.

31. Leonard, J. M., Bremmer, W. J., Capell, P. T., and Paulsen, C. A.: Male hypogonadism: Klinefelter and Reifenstein syndromes. *In* Bergsma, D. (ed.): National Foundation. Birth Defects Original Article Series, Genetic Forms of Hypogonadism 1975, p. 17–22.

32. Levy, E. P., Pashayan, H., Fraser, F. C., and Pinsky, L.: XX and XY Turner phenotypes in a family. Amer. J. Dis. Child., *120*:36, 1970.

33. Lubs, H. A., Jr., Vilar, O., and Bergenstal, D. M.: Familial male pseudohermaphroditism with labial testes and partial feminization: endocrine studies and genetic aspects. J. Clin. Endocrinol. Metab., *19*:1110, 1959.

34. Madden, J. D., Walsh, P. C., MacDonald, P. C., and Wilson, J. D.: Clinical and endocrinological characterization of a patient with the syndrome of incomplete testicular feminization. J. Clin. Endocrinol. Metab., *1*:751, 1975.

35. Molitor, J. T., Chertoio, B. S., and Fariss, B. L.: Long-term follow-up of a patient with congenital adrenal hyperplasia and failure of testicular development. Fertil. Steril., *24*:319, 1973.

36. Mortimer, C. H., McNeilly, A. S., Fisher, R. A., Murray, M. A. F., and Besser, G. M.: Gonadotropin-releasing hormone therapy in hypogonadal males with hypothalamic or pituitary dysfunction. Brit. Med. J., 4:617, 1974.
37. Naftolin, F., Harris, G. W., and Bobrow, J. W.: Effect of purified luteinizing hormone releasing factor on normal and hypogonadotropic anosmic men. Nature, 232:496, 1971.
38. Nasr, H., Chen, J. C., Pearson, O. H., and Wieland, R. G.: Chromatin-negative Klinefelter's syndrome with normal testes and serum gonadotropins and testosterone. Fertil. Steril., 2:761, 1971.
39. New, M. I.: Male pseudohermaphroditism due to 17α-hydroxylase deficiency. J. Clin. Invest., 49:1930, 1970.
40. Odell, W. D. and Swerdloff, R. S.: Male hypogonadism. West. J. Med., 124:446, 1976.
41. Pasqualini, R. Q., and Bur, G. E.: Sindrome hipandrogenico con gametogenesis conservada: Clarificacion de la insuficiencia testicular. Rev. Asoc. Med. Argent., 64:6, 1950.
42. Paulsen, C. A.: The testes. In Williams, R. H. (ed.): Textbook of Endocrinology, 5th ed. Philadelphia, W. B. Saunders Co., 1974, p. 323–367.
43. Paulsen, C. A., Gordon, D. L., Carpenter, R. W., Gandy, H. M., and Drucker, W. D.: Klinefelter's syndrome and its variants: a hormonal and chromosomal study. Recent Progr. Horm. Res., 24:321, 1968.
44. Phadke, A. G., MacKinnon, K. J., and Dossetor, J. B.: Male fertility in uremia: restoration by renal allografts. Can. Med. Assoc. J. 102:607, 1970.
45. Plymate, S. R,, Bremner, W. J., and Paulsen, C. A.: The association of D-group chromosomal translocations and defective spermatogenesis. Fertil. Steril., 27:139, 1976.
46. Prader, A., Zachmann, M., and Illig, R.: Normal spermatogenesis in adult males with congenital adrenal hyperplasia after discontinuation of therapy. In Lee, P. A., Platnick, L., Kowarski, A. A., and Migeon, C. J. (eds.): Congenital Adrenal Hyperplasia, Baltimore, University Park Press, in press.
47. Rabin, D., Spitz, I., Bercovici, B., et al.: Isolated deficiency of follicle-stimulating hormone. N. Engl. J. Med., 287:1313, 1972.
48. Radfar, R., Bartter, F. C., Easley, R., Kolins, J., and Sherins, R. J.: Evidence for endogenous LH suppression in a man with bilateral testicular tumors and congenital adrenal hyperplasia. J. Clin. Endocrinol. Metab., in press.
49. Reifenstein, E. C., Jr.: Hereditary familial hypogonadism. Clin. Res., 3:86, 1947.
50. Rosewater, S., Gwinup, G., and Hamwi, G. J.: Familial gynecomastia. Ann. Intern. Med., 63:377, 1965.
51. Santen, R. J., Leonard, J. M., Shernins, R. J., Gandy, H. M., and Paulsen, C. A.: Short and long-term effects of clomiphene citrate on the pituitary-testicular axis. J. Clin. Endocrinol., 33:970, 1971.
52. Santen, R. J., and Paulsen, C. A.: Hypogonadotropic eunuchoidism, I. Clinical study of the mode of inheritance. J. Clin. Endocrinol. Metab., 36:47, 1973.
53. Santen, R. J., and Paulsen, C. A.: Hypogonadotropic eunuchoidism, II. Gonadal responsiveness to exogenous gonadotropin. J. Clin. Endocrinol. Metab., 36:55, 1973.
54. Schalch, D. S., Gonzalez-Barcena, D., Kastin, A. J., Landa, L., Lee, L. A., Zamora, M. T., and Schally, A. V.: Plasma gonadotropins after administration of LH-releasing hormone in patients with renal or hepatic failure. J. Clin. Endocrinol. Metab., 41:921, 1975.
55. Schneider, G., Genel, M., Bongiovanni, A. M., Goldman, A. S., and Rosenfield, R. L.: Persistent testicular $\Delta^{5=}$isomerase-3β-hydroxysteroid dehydrogenase (Δ^5-3β-HSD) deficiency in the Δ^5-3β-HSD form of congenital adrenal hyperplasia. J. Clin. Invest., 55:581, 1975.
56. Stewart-Bentley, M., Gans, D., and Horton, R.: Regulation of gonadal function in uremia. Metabolism, 23:1065, 1974.
57. Wachtel, S. S., Koo, G. C., Breg, W. R., et al.: Serologic detection of a Y-linked gene in XX males and XX true hermaphrodites. N. Engl. J. Med., 295:750, 1976.
58. Walsh, P. C.: Physiologic basis for hormonal therapy in carcinoma of the prostate. Urol. Clin. N. Amer., 2:125, 1975.
59. Walsh, P. C., Madden, J. D., Harrod, M. J., Goldstein, J. L., MacDonald, P. C., and Wilson, J. D.: Familial incomplete male pseudohermaphroditism, type 2. Decreased

dihydrotestosterone formation in pseudovaginal perineoscrotal hypospadias. N. Engl. J. Med., *291*:944, 1974.

60. Walsh, P. C., and Swerdloff, R. S.: Biphasic effect of testosterone on spermatogenesis in the rat. Invest. Urol., *11*:190, 1973.

61. Wiener, S., Sutherland, G., Bartholomew, A. A., and Hudson, B.: XYY males in a Melbourne prison. Lancet, *1*:150, 1968.

62. Wilson, J. D., Harrod, M. J., Goldstein, J. L., Hemsell, D. L., and MacDonald, P. C.: Familial incomplete male pseudohermaphroditism, type 1. Evidence for androgen resistance and variable clinical manifestations in a family with the Reifenstein's syndrome. N. Engl. J. Med., *290*:1097, 1974.

63. Wilson, J. D., and MacDonald, P. C.: Male pseudohermaphroditism due to androgen resistance: testicular feminization and related syndromes. In Stanbury, J. B., Wyngaarden, J., and Fredericksen, D. S. Metabolic Basis of Inherited Disease. New York, McGraw-Hill Book Co., in press.

64. Winter, J. S. D., Taraska, S., and Faiman, C.: The hormonal response to HCG stimulation in male children and adolescents. J. Clin. Endocrinol. Metab., *34*:348, 1972.

65. Wong, T. W., Straus, F. H., and Warner, N. E.: Testicular biopsy in the study of male infertility. III. Pretesticular causes of infertility. Arch. Pathol., *98*:1, 1974.

66. Zachman, M., Vollmin, J. A., Hamilton, W., and Prader, A.: Steroid 17,20-desmolase deficiency: a new cause of male pseudohermaphroditism. Clin. Endocrinol., *1*:369, 1972.

Chapter 3

THE VARICOCELE
AND INFERTILITY

Lawrence Dubin, M.D.
Richard D. Amelar, M.D.

INTRODUCTION

Varicocele is a well-established cause of male infertility. Of 1294 consecutive cases of male infertility seen from 1965 to 1970, we found 39 per cent to be caused by varicocele.[11] Although this figure may be high because of our interest in this problem, other authors have confirmed that the incidence is significant and deserves attention in the diagnosis and therapy of male fertility problems.[2-4, 16, 26, 29]

The deleterious effect of varicocele as related to fertility was well established in an article by Johnson *et al.* in 1970.[21] In routine physical examinations for military induction performed on 1592 young males, 9.5 per cent (151 men) had asymptomatic varicocele. Ninety-three agreed to have a semen analysis performed, and 63 of these had significant semen abnormalities.

HISTORICAL ASPECTS

Varicocele was noted as a cause of male infertility as early as the 1880s by a British surgeon named Barfield.[34] In 1929 Macomber and Sand-

57

ers reported restoration of fertility in men following bilateral varicocele surgery.[23] However, it was not until Tulloch's report in 1952[32] of restored spermatogenesis in an azoospermic man with varicocele that real notice was taken of the problem. It is significant that in general therapeutic results in azoospermic men since that time have been poor.[14, 24, 28] Since Tulloch's work in the 1950s numerous reports of success following varicocele ligation have appeared in the literature. The major reports are listed in Table 3-1.[2, 3]

The seminal picture seen in subfertile men with varicocele was described in 1965 by MacLeod.[22] Oligospermia of varying degrees was noted, but of more importance were the signs of a marked impairment of sperm motility and a definite increase of immature and tapering sperm forms in the ejaculum. Indeed, although the sperm count frequently improves following ligation of the varicocele, the response is often limited to an improvement in sperm motility and a decrease in immature sperm forms.

Dubin and Hotchkiss in 1969[14] studied testicular biopsies from subfertile men with varicocele and found germinal cell hypoplasia and a premature sloughing of immature sperm forms within the lumina of the seminiferous tubules. These cells were similar to those seen in the ejaculum and included tapering forms and spermatids in a stage between Clermont Sb–1 and Sb–2[19] (see Figs. 3–1 and 3–2). On testicular histology varicoceles showed no preference for the right or left side. Those patients who did not improve showed no specific histologic pattern.

ETIOLOGY

The cause of varicocele as a source of male infertility has not been completely elucidated. Hanley and Harrison (1956) suggested that the ef-

Table 3–1 SPERMATOGENESIS FOLLOWING
LIGATION OF VARICOCELE

INVESTIGATOR	NO. PATIENTS	SEMEN IMPROVEMENT (%)	PREGNANCY (%)
Tulloch, 1955[33]	30	66	Not reported
Charny, 1962[7]	36	64	30
Scott and Young,[27] 1962	166	70	Not reported
Hanley and Harrison,[18] 1962	60	70	30
Brown, MacLeod, and Hotchkiss,[6] 1968	185	55 to 60	43
Dubin and Amelar,[10] 1970	111	81	48
Stewart,[28] 1974	20	85	55
Dubin and Amelar,[12, 13] 1975	504	71	55

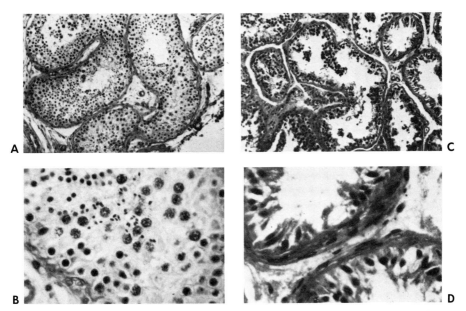

Figure 3-1. Testis biopsies. *A*. Normal testis. (100 ×) *B*. Normal testis. (450 ×) *C*. Biopsy from subfertile man with variococele. (100 ×) *D*, Biopsy from subfertile man with varicocele. (450 ×).

fect was secondary to increased heat in the scrotum caused by stasis of blood.[17] This, however, has been disputed in other studies by Tessler and Krahn in 1966.[31]

Zorgniotti and MacLeod[35] reported in 1973 that the intrascrotal temperature in 50 oligospermic men with varicocele was an average of 0.6° C.

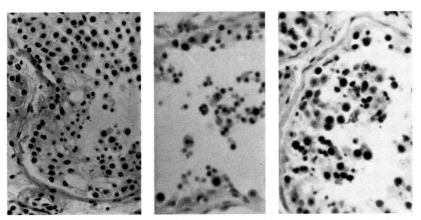

Figure 3-2. Testis biopsies, showing premature sloughing of immature cells into lumina of tubules. *Left*, normal male after treatment with antispermatogenic drug. *Center* and *right*, biopsies from subfertile men with varicocele. (450 ×)

higher than that in a control group of 35 medical students with normal semen. Some oligospermic men without palpable varicocele had abnormal intrascrotal temperatures similar to those in men with varicocele. There is a possibility that this was caused by clinically undetectable retrograde blood flow in the left internal spermatic vein. Most recently, in 1976 Comhaire et al.[8] found abnormal thermograms in 37 of 39 oligospermic men with varicocele. Among 36 men suspected of having subclinical varicocele, 19 had abnormal thermograms, and 16 of these showed reflux in the left internal spermatic vein on venography.

Swerdloff and Walsh[30] studied 13 subfertile men with clinical varicocele. The levels of luteinizing hormone (LH), follicle-stimulating hormone (FSH), testosterone and estradiol in the peripheral veins were obtained, as were the levels of testosterone and estradiol in the internal spermatic vein. Secretion of both gonadal steroids and pituitary gonadotropins was normal. It appears likely that mechanisms other than abnormal reproductive hormonal factors are responsible for the poor quality of the semen in these patients.

Another theory became more acceptable when the rich anastomoses of the veins of the pampiniform plexus between the venous drainage of the left and right testicles were demonstrated.[15] Due to venous valvular incompetence, the blood flows in a retrograde manner down the left internal spermatic vein in patients with varicocele.[5] It has been shown radiographically, using radiopaque contrast media injected into the internal spermatic vein, that the blood on the left side in the man with varicocele mixes with that on the right side, allowing for an adverse effect on the two sides.[4]

By injecting radiopaque dye directly into the left renal vein via catheter, it has also been shown that the blood from the left renal vein can flow in a retrograde manner along the left internal spermatic vein in patients with varicocele.[1] It is believed that blood from the left adrenal and left renal veins carrying a relatively high concentration of toxic metabolic substances such as steroids, which are potential spermatogenic inhibitors, can enter the left internal spermatic vein directly and in an undetoxified state; these "toxins" can reach both testicles and affect sperm production. Comhaire and Vermeulen have hypothesized that chronic testicular exposure to catecholamine-rich blood might explain the disturbance in spermatogenesis found in these patients.[9]

Varicocele usually occurs on the left side owing to the insertion of the left internal spermatic vein into the renal vein at a right angle; the right internal spermatic vein usually enters the inferior vena cava at an oblique angle. Man's erect posture may contribute to the increased pressure in the venous system. In addition, the superior mesenteric artery and aorta may squeeze the left renal vein while beating in synchrony, causing increased pressure on the valves at the junction of the internal spermatic and left renal veins.

If this theory of blood toxins and retrograde venous flow is correct, then the solution to the problem of male infertility is ligation of the left internal spermatic vein at a point above the cross-over anastomosis with the venous drainage from the right testicle. If this is done surgically at or above the level of the internal inguinal ring, the venous drainage from the left testicle will take the routes of the uninterrupted external spermatic and deferential veins. This theory implies that varicocele itself is a result of retrograde venous blood flow in the internal spermatic veins rather than a cause of male infertility. This concept has been corroborated by recent studies showing that the size of varicocele preoperatively has no effect on the results of ligation of the internal spermatic vein.[10] The results in improved semen quality and increase in pregnancies were just as good regardless of whether the varicocele was judged preoperatively to be large, moderate, or small.

DIAGNOSIS

Diagnosis of varicocele is not always a simple matter. The patient must be examined in the upright position, since all but large varicoceles will be missed if the patient is in the recumbent position owing to venous decompression. Reflux of blood into the scrotum should be determined by manual palpation with the patient performing the Valsalva maneuver (see Chapter 6). This maneuver is extremely important because small varicoceles will not be diagnosed without it and the correct therapy will therefore not be instituted.

Using this diagnostic maneuver, bilateral varicoceles have been diagnosed in 14 per cent of 504 of our subfertile patients.[12, 13] Injection techniques have suggested that in these men the right internal spermatic vein has an anomalous anatomic relationship in that, as on the left side, it enters directly into the right renal vein rather than obliquely into the vena cava as it usually does on the right side.

These 504 men were studied over a 10-year period (1963 to 1973). High ligation of the internal spermatic vein was performed in all cases. They had good follow-up for at least 1 year after varicocelectomy.

All patients were evaluated preoperatively and had normal thyroid, adrenocortical, and pituitary gonadotropin function. At least two semen specimens from each patient were checked prior to surgery; all specimens showed varying amounts of oligospermia, severely impaired sperm motility, and an increase in immature and tapering forms in the ejaculate. Azoospermic patients were eliminated from the study.

All patients had tried unsuccessfully to produce a pregnancy for at least 1 year prior to evaluaiton, and many had received previous therapy with medications elsewhere. The results of the reported study are shown in Table 3–2.

Table 3–2 RESULTS IN 504 MEN BEFORE AND AFTER VARICOCELECTOMY, WITH OR WITHOUT HUMAN CHORIONIC GONADOTROPIN THERAPY*

			PREOPERATIVE OLIGOSPERMIC SPERM COUNTS						
			<10 mill/ml[a]				*>10 mill/ml. (No HCG Therapy)*	
	Total		*No HCG Therapy*		*HCG Therapy[b]*			
PATIENTS AND WIVES	*No.*	*%*	*No.*	*%*	*No.*	*%*	*No.*	*%*
Total number	504	—	123	—	50	—	331	—
Number with improved semen quality	361	70	41	33	28	56	292	88
Number of pregnancies	276	55	28	23	22	44	226	68

*Dubin, L., and Amelar, R. D.: Varicocelectomy as therapy in male infertility: A study of 504 cases. Fertil. Steril.. 26:217, 1975.

[a]Not azoospermic.

[b]80,000 units given over a 10-week period after varicocelectomy.

SEMEN QUALITY

Of the 504 patients studied, 431 (85.5 per cent) had left-sided varicoceles only; 71 (14 per cent) had bilateral varicoceles and underwent bilateral varicocelectomy. Two patients had right-sided varicocelectomy only; one of these had situs inversus, while the other had previously undergone left orchiectomy.

After surgery, 361 (71 per cent) patients had a marked improvement in semen quality, and 276 (55 per cent) of their wives became pregnant (Table 3–2).

Of the 331 men who had preoperative sperm counts of over 10 million per ml. (Table 3–2), 292 (88 per cent) had improved semen quality resulting in 226 (68 per cent) pregnancies.

Of the 173 men who had preoperative sperm counts of less than 10 million per ml., 123 had no additional therapy; 41 (33 per cent) of these had improved semen quality with 28 (23 per cent) resultant pregnancies.

In an effort to improve on these results, 50 of the patients with preoperative sperm counts of less than 10 million per ml. were treated empirically with varicocelectomy and postoperative human chorionic gonadotropin (80,000 units) over a 10-week period. Twenty-eight (56 per cent) men showed improved semen quality, resulting in 22 (44 per cent) pregnancies (Table 3–2).

The 276 pregnancies occurred at a mean of 5.5 months and a median of 6.7 months after varicocelectomy (Table 3–3). Two hundred and seventeen patients' wives delivered 220 babies; 117 infants (53 per cent) were female and 103 (47 per cent) were male. There were three sets of twins. Twelve miscarriages and two ectopic pregnancies occurred. Forty-five wives were still pregnant at the time of writing. Some of the patients fathered more than one child after varicocelectomy: 30 had two children, eight had three children, and one had four children.

The relatively few postoperative complications (Table 3–4) attest to the benign nature of the surgery.

Recurrence of the varicocele occurred in one patient. This patient and his wife had been trying for a pregnancy for 4 years. The patient's initial sperm count was over 10 million per ml., but semen quality was poor. A left varicocelectomy was performed on February 10, 1966; semen quality improved, and pregnancy occurred 12 months after surgery. A son was born on November 9, 1967. Difficulty in achieving a second pregnancy and poor semen quality were noted again 3 years after surgery. Examination revealed that the varicocele had recurred. Reflux of blood was again noted during scrotal palpation using the Valsalva maneuver. A second operation was performed, and a large single internal spermatic vein was ligated. Postoperatively, a marked improvement in semen quality was noted, and pregnancy occurred 3 months after surgery. A daughter was born on August 10, 1970. A third pregnancy then occurred, and another son was born on January 6, 1972.

Table 3-3 TIME BETWEEN VARICOCELECTOMY OF PATIENT AND PREGNANCY OF WIFE

MONTH	NO. PREGNANCIES
1	0
2	11
3	55
4	38
5	27
6	29
7	23
8	18
9	10
10	16
11	11
12	12
13	8
14	3
15	3
16	2
17	2
18	5
19	0
20	1
21	0
22	1
23	1
Total	276

5.5 Mean (months)
6.7 Median (months)

Seventeen (3 per cent) patients had hydrocele formation postoperatively. The exact cause of this is unknown, but the low incidence is probably related to careful ligation of the veins alone with preservation of all lymphatic channels. Three patients required operative hydrocelectomy.

Table 3-4 POSTOPERATIVE COMPLICATIONS FROM VARICOCELECTOMY IN 504 MEN

COMPLICATION	NO. MEN
Hydrocele not requiring hydrocelectomy	14
Hydrocele requiring hydrocelectomy	3
Wound infection	4
Inguinal hematoma	2
Left epididymitis	1
Atelectasis	1
Recurrence of varicocele	1

SURGICAL TREATMENT OF VARICOCELE

The major problem in varicocele seems to be retrograde blood flow from the renal vein into the scrotal circulation secondary to incompetent valves in the internal spermatic venous system. The problem can be corrected by interrupting the course of the internal spermatic vein to prevent retrograde flow rather than by removing the dilated scrotal veins. Three approaches are available as described in the following paragraphs.

Ivanissevich Procedure[20] (modified by Amelar and Dubin) (Fig. 3–3). An inguinal incision is made over the area of the internal inguinal ring. The external oblique muscle is incised through the external inguinal ring, and a self-retaining retractor is placed in the wound. The spermatic cord is dissected free. A Penrose drain is then placed under the spermatic cord and the cord is lifted out of the incision by the drain, which is then clamped on each end to the drapes. The external spermatic fascia is incised, and the veins are dissected free while trying to preserve all lymphatic channels. The internal spermatic veins are then ligated and partially excised at the internal inguinal ring. Usually two or three branches of the internal spermatic vein are located in this area. The spermatic cord is returned to its position, and the external oblique fascia is closed with 2–0 chromic catgut. The skin is closed with interrupted silk or nylon sutures. No drains are used.

Palomo Procedure.[25] An inguinal incision similar to that used in the Ivanissevich procedure but slightly higher and extended through the external oblique muscle is made. An incision is then made in the internal oblique fascia in the direction of the muscle fibers approximately 2 inches above the internal ring. The internal oblique fascia is spread apart, and retroperitoneal dissection is performed; this usually exposes two branches of the internal spermatic vein, which are then ligated and incised. The internal oblique is then closed with 2–0 chromic catgut, and the remainder of the closure proceeds as described previously.

Scrotal Approach. The transcrotal approach, which utilizes multiple clamping and ligation of the numerous vessels of the pampiniform plexus, is not recommended because many veins may be missed and end–artery damage at this level is a danger. Scrotal swelling and hematoma may also lead to delayed recovery of fertility.

We favor the Amelar and Dubin modification of the Ivanissevich procedure. It is simple and can be done well by the average surgeon, and results have been excellent.

Many questions about the actual effects of varicocele on fertility still remain unanswered. First, many men with varicocele have normal semen qualities and adequate fertility. Second, the actual toxic metabolic substance in the refluxing blood has not been definitely identified. Third, a study of varicocelectomy failures (which represent 20 to 30 per cent of all patients reported) does not reveal any preoperative differences from the group that showed improvement. Nevertheless, the good results in semen

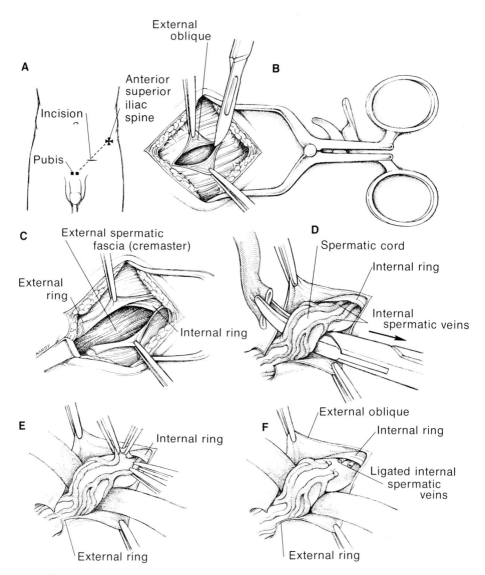

Figure 3–3. Varicocelectomy (Ivanissevich procedure modified by Amelar and Dubin). *A.* An inguinal incision is made over the area of the internal inguinal ring. *B* and *C.* An incision is made in the external oblique muscle extending through the external inguinal ring, and a self-retaining retractor is placed in the wound. *D.* The spermatic cord is dissected free. A Penrose drain is then placed under the spermatic cord. *E* and *F.* The internal spermatic veins are then dissected while attempting to preserve all lymphatic channels. The veins are then interrupted, ligated, and partially excised at the internal inguinal ring.

improvement and pregnancy rate continue to make this form of therapy one of the most effective in the treatment of male infertility.

REFERENCES

1. Ahlberg, N. E., Bartley, O., and Chidekel, N.: Retrograde contrast filling of the left gonadal vein: a roentgenologic and anatomical study. Acta Radiol. (Diag.), 3:385, 1965.
2. Amelar, R. D., and Dubin, L.: Male infertility, current diagnosis and treatment. Urology, 1:1, 1973.
3. Amelar, R. D., and Dubin, L.: Basic and practical aspects of the etiology and management of male infertility. Urol. Digest, 14:19, 1975.
4. Brown, J. S., Dubin, L., Becker, M., and Hotchkiss, R. S.: Venography in the subfertile man with varicocele. J. Urol., 98:388, 1967.
5. Brown, J. S., Dubin, L., and Hotchkiss, R. S.: Varicocele as related to fertility. Fertil. Steril., 18:46, 1967.
6. Brown, J. S., MacLeod, J., and Hotchkiss, R. S.: Results of varicocelectomy in subfertile men. Exhibit at American Fertility Society, Miami, Florida, 1968.
7. Charny, C. W.: Effect of varicocele on fertility. Fertil. Steril., 13:47, 1962.
8. Comhaire, F., Monteyner, R., and Kunnen, M.: The value of scrotal thermography as compared with selective retrograde venography of the internal spermatic vein for the diagnosis of subclinical varicocele. Fertil. Steril., 27:694, 1976.
9. Comhaire, F., and Vermeulen, A.: Varicocele sterility; cortisol and catecholamines. Fertil. Steril., 25:88, 1974.
10. Dubin, L., and Amelar, R. D.: Varicocele size and results of varicocelectomy in selected subfertile men with varicocele. Fertil. Steril., 21:606, 1970.
11. Dubin, L., and Amelar, R. D.: Etiologic factors in 1294 consecutive cases of male infertility. Fertil. Steril., 22:469, 1971.
12. Dubin, L., and Amelar, R. D.: Varicocelectomy as therapy in male infertility: A study of 504 cases. Fertil. Steril., 26:217, 1975.
13. Dubin, L., and Amelar, R. D.: Varcocelectomy as therapy in male infertility. J. Urol., 113:(5) 640, 1975.
14. Dubin, L., and Hotchkiss, R. S.: Testis biopsy in subfertile men with varicocele. Fertil. Steril., 20:50, 1969.
15. El-Sadr, A. R., and Mina, E.: Anatomical and surgical aspects in operative management of varicocele. Urol. Cutan. Rev., 54:257, 1950.
16. Hamen, R.: Studies on Impaired Fertility in Men, with Special Reference to the Male. London, Oxford University Press, 1944, pp. 22, 108.
17. Hanley, H. G.: The surgery of male sub-fertility. Ann. R. Coll. Surg. Eng., 17:159, 1955.
18. Hanley, H. G., and Harrison, R. G.: Nature and surgical correction of varicocele. Br. J. Surg., 50:64, 1962.
19. Heller, C. G., and Clermont, Y.: Kinetics of the germinal epithelium in man. Prog. Horm. Res., 20:545, 1964.
20 Ivanissevich, O.: Left varicocele due to reflux, experience with 4470 operatives cases in 42 years. J. Int. Coll. Surg., 24:742, 1960.
21. Johnson, D., Pohl, D., and Rivera-Correa, H.: Varicocele: an innocuous condition? South. Med. J., 63:34, 1970.
22. MacLeod, J.: Seminal cytology in the presence of varicocele. Fertil. Steril., 16:735, 1965.
23. Macomber, D., and Sanders, M. D.: The spermatozoa count. N. Engl. J. Med., 200:981, 1929.
24. Mehan, D. J.: Results of ligation of internal spermatic vein in the treatment of infertility in azoospermic patients. Fertil. Steril., 27:110, 1976.
25. Palomo, A.: Radical cure of varicocele by a new technique. J. Urol., 61:604, 1949.
26. Russell, J. K.: Varicocele in groups of fertile and subfertile men. Br. Med. J., 1:1231, 1954.
27. Scott, L. S., and Young, D.: Varicocele. Fertil. Steril., 13:325, 1962.
28. Stewart, B.: Varicocele in infertility: incidence and results of surgical therapy. J. Urol., 112:222, 1974.

29. Stewart, B., and Montie, J.: Male infertility, an optimistic report. J. Urol., *110*:216, 1973.
30. Swerdloff, R. S., and Walsh, P.: Pituitary gonadal hormones in patients with varicocele. Fertil. Steril., *26*:1006, 1975.
31. Tessler, A. N., and Krahn, H. P.: Varicocele and testicular temperature. Fertil. Steril., *17*:201, 1966.
32. Tulloch, W. S.: Consideration of sterility; subfertility in the male. Edinburgh Med. J., *59*:29, 1952.
33. Tulloch, W. S.: Varicocele in subfertility: results of treatment. Br. Med. J., *2*:356, 1955.
34. Zorgniotti, A. W.: The spermatozoa count, a short history. Urology, *5*:672, 1975.
35. Zorgniotti, A. W., and MacLeod, J.: Studies in temperature, human semen quality and varicocele. Fertil. Steril., *24*:854, 1973.

Chapter 4

OTHER FACTORS AFFECTING MALE FERTILITY

RICHARD D. AMELAR, M.D.
LAWRENCE DUBIN, M.D.

Various factors may interrupt or alter the orderly progression of maturation of the sperm cells and cause infertility. In general, the spermatogenic cells appear to become increasingly sensitive to toxic agents as they develop. Thus, spermatids appear to be the most sensitive and spermatogonia the least sensitive, except to irradiation, in which the sequence is reversed. Sertoli cells are the most resistant among all the elements of the germinal epithelium. It should also be noted that injury to the germinal epithelium is often not uniformly distributed throughout the testes; some tubules may show extensive damage, whereas others appear to remain essentially normal.

The Leydig, or interstitial, cells, which produce male hormones, lie completely outside the seminiferous tubules and are not affected by heat and drugs that may have a deleterious effect upon the germinal epithelium. It is worth emphasizing to the infertile husband that the testicles have two separate functions, production of sperm and production of hormones, and that it is possible to be completely masculine from a hormonal and personality point of view even though sperm production may be deficient or absent.

During the orderly, step by step maturation process of spermatogenesis mature sperm accumulate at the central lumen of the seminiferous tubule and are then, in a continuous process, shed into the lumen and conducted to the efferent canals of the rete testis and then to the epididymis; finally, they pass through the ductal system where they are stored prior to ejaculation. During this process several factors may affect sperm production and delivery; apart from endocrinologic factors (Chapter 2) and varicocele (Chapter 3), these factors are considered in this chapter.

ALTITUDE AND CLIMATE

High altitude is known to affect testicular function and fertility adversely. The effect of this unfavorable environment on fertility may be illustrated by the Spanish conquerors of Bolivia who founded the city of Potosi 14,000 feet above sea level. Here 100,000 natives continued to reproduce as usual, but the Spaniards either did not succeed in having children or produced children who failed to survive. The birth of the first viable baby among the Spaniards did not take place until 53 years after the founding of the city and was attributed to a miracle performed by St. Nicholas of Tolentino.[29]

According to the Foundation Charter of Lima, the captial of Peru was transferred in 1535 from Jauja (11,500 feet above sea level) to Lima (at sea level) because horses and pigs did not reproduce in Jauja. It was found that male cats and rabbits became azoospermic when transferred to Morococha, 14,000 feet above sea level in the Andes, and that the germinal epithelium of these animals contained only spermatogonia and Sertoli cells.[121]

Among the most effective inhibitors of sperm production is transfer to a hot climate, especially when it has relatively high humidity. It is a common observation that farm animals transferred from a temperate climate to moist hot tropics are slow in reproducing, and the same may be true of the human male.[65] When mice are placed in an atmosphere of high humidity at 37° C., the males at once stop producing sperm and become sterile; however, after a time the mice become tolerant of the heat and resume spermatogenesis.[195] Like mice, large domestic animals also develop tolerance to heat slowly and gradually increase their fertility.

HEAT

Elevation of the testicular temperature to the level of body temperature in most mammals (elephants, rhinoceris and whales are exceptions) is injurious to testicular activity.[53, 182, 202] Hence, nature provides that the testes are carried outside the body in the scrotal sac. It has been amply proved that a testicular temperature lower by 4° to 5° F. than the body temperature is essential for spermatogenesis. The human testicles, situated in the scrotum, lie in an environment that is cooler by an average of 2.2°C. than the intra-abdominal temperature.[13, 129] If the testicles are exposed for any significant length of time to temperatures at or higher than body temperature, maturation ceases at the secondary spermatocyte stage, and the sperm count will drop in proportion to the number of tubules affected. The interstitial, or Leydig, cells outside the tubules are not affected by temperature changes and continue to produce hormone. Arrest of the sperm maturation process by heat is generally completely reversible; if the heat is diminished, the sperm count may be restored to normal within 3 months.

Possible sources of heat that may affect spermatogenesis are a febrile illness, prolonged and frequent hot baths, and tight undergarments such as athletic supporters that may hold the scrotum close to the body, thus interfering with scrotal ventilation.[145, 147] Studies on the effect of hydrocele on the scrotum[86] showed no significant increase in scrotal temperature and no effect on spermatogenesis due to the presence of a hydrocele. Hence, the possibility of diminished spermatogenesis cannot be used as a reasonable argument in favor of treating a hydrocele.

FEBRILE ILLNESS

Frequently one finds a temporarily poor semen specimen as the result of an acute febrile illness. Studies on volunteers subjected to fever induction[110] showed that low levels in sperm cell counts were reached at 25 to 55 days after the treatment and continued for 15 to 50 days; this was followed by a recovery period lasting from 25 to 30 days. Full recovery occurred within 3 months in every case. This was the first study demonstrating that induced hyperpyrexia does depress sperm output in humans. There is also documentation of reduced sperm output in such febrile illnesses as pneumonia[106] and in the recurrent febrile attacks of familial Mediterranean fever.[50]

It has been observed that acute viral illnesses such as mononucleosis, chickenpox, and hepatitis can also cause temporary but often marked depression of sperm production.[5, 106] When evaluating a poor semen specimen it is therefore important to know whether the man has had a febrile illness within the previous 3 months. Since the deleterious effects of hyperthermia on spermatogenesis will be completely dissipated after 3 months, it is best to repeat the semen analysis 3 months after elimination of the increased heat to the testicles.

Cold is evidently much less damaging to spermatogenesis than heat; however, severe chilling of the testes, as with the application of ice packs, can produce decapitation of epididymal sperm and destruction of the spermatogenic epithelium.[30, 64, 105]

In our own clinical experience with therapy of oligospermic men, we have found no beneficial effects from the use of alternating hot and cold applications to the testes as advocated by Robinson and Rock.[146] Similarly, we have not seen any benefit to patients who have poor semen quality merely from exchanging tight "jockey" type undershorts for looser fitting "boxer" type undershorts.

CRYPTORCHISM

A notable instance of the irreversible effect of heat on spermatogenesis occurs in the cryptorchid child with *late descent of one or both testes.* Here it has been demonstrated that if the child's testicle remains outside of the scrotum after the age of 5 years, irreversible[31, 66] changes begin to take place, and if the testicle remains outside of the scrotum until puberty, it will be incapable of producing sperm thereafter. Cryptorchism should therefore be corrected by the age of 5 years. The chances of preserving fertility are decreased the longer the correction is delayed toward puberty.[4, 56, 168]

In discussing cryptorchism, it is important to distinguish between the two main groups of undescended testes—*retractile* and *true maldescended testes.* Scorer and Farrington[167] have pointed out that the retractile testis, which is due to a hyperactive cremasteric reflex, will descend by puberty as maturation occurs. The incidence of cryptorchism at the age of 1 year is 0.2 to 0.7 per cent, the same as that in the adult population. However, at age 5 to 6, the incidence is more than double that seen in the adult. Consequently, most of the patients with undescended testes seen at this age have retractile testes. Scorer[166] estimates that approximately two thirds of children examined for unilateral testicular maldescent have this type of retractile testis rather than a true maldescended testicle.

Of the remaining third of all cases of unilateral cryptorchism, about 80 per cent are classified as *obstructed testes.* The obstructed testis usually lies in the superficial inguinal pouch or superficial to the external oblique aponeurosis. It has good cord length and is grossly normal to inspection.

The remaining 20 per cent of these nonretractile testes are *functionally dystopic* and may be located high in the scrotum, within the inguinal canal, or intra-abdominally, or they may be congenitally absent.

Cryptorchism associated with *true testicular ectopia* is extremely rare (affecting less than 1 per cent of all nonretractile cryptochid testes). These ectopic testes lie outside the route of normal testicular descent — i.e., in the perineum or the femoral region or in front of the symphysis pubis.

The retractile testicle will often respond to medical management with injections of human chorionic gonadotropin, but the nonretractile maldescended testicle must be treated surgically.

In the past it has been generally assumed that one normally positioned testis is adequate for good fertility potential and that unilateral cryptorchism should not present the problem of impaired semen quality. However, a recent retrospective study[99] indicates that there may be an intrinsic defect in testicular tissue in the dystopic testis, and in patients with unilateral cryptorchism the scrotal testis may also be abnormal. Studies by Minenberg and Bingol indicate that the defect may be on a chromosomal level and that it may be associated with an increased proclivity toward malignant disease.[120]

Lipshultz *et al.* carried out a retrospective study on 29 patients who had had surgical correction of cryptorchism 20 years ago.[99] The mean age at the time of surgery in this group was 8.6 years. The patient's were compared with an age-matched group of controls. Semen analyses demonstrated that the mean sperm density for the control group was 73.6 million sperm per ml., whereas that of the post-unilateral orchiopexy group was only 26.8 million per ml. Furthermore, 11 of the 29 patients in the latter group had sperm densities of less than 20 million per ml.

Despite these findings, Lipshultz[98] feels that it is important to place the dystopic testis in the scrotum before the age of 5 years, even if there is an inherited defect in testicular tissue in these cases. Although the inherited defect may not be reversible, the additional deleterious effect of the extrascrotal position may be reversible or at least "arrestable," and some spermatogenic function may be preserved for future fertility.

Thus, orchiopexy before age 5 is advisable to ensure minimal histologic changes that may be secondary to the testis' increased exposure to elevated extrascrotal temperatures. Surgical correction is advised when human chorionic gonadotropin stimulation fails to produce testicular descent, thereby defining the maldescended testicle as truly "cryptorchid" and not merely retractile.

The details of the management of cryptorchism by hormonal or surgical treatment are described in Chapter 11.

STRESS AND EMOTIONAL FACTORS

It is well known that psychogenic factors can affect a man's sexual performance and therefore his ability to deliver his sperm into the vagina.

In general, stress, anxiety, and emotional tension can also have deleterious effects on sperm production. This is not unexpected considering the role of the hypothalamus, which is located between the cerebral cortex and the hypophysis and is the source of the neurohumoral-releasing factors that are now known to control gonadotropin release from the pituitary. Emotional stress or disturbance will alter hypothalamic function; this in turn will lead to failure of gonadotropin-releasing factors to act on the pituitary, and thus may result in hypothalamic hypogonadotropism. To affect fertility, however, the stress involved must be of extreme proportions, and the ordinary pressures of life and work have not in our experience been sufficient to cause male infertility.

The first documented work on the effect of stress on human spermatogenesis was a study by Sand in 1933 of prisoners sentenced to death who were kept waiting a long time before the sentence was executed.[160] Severe, progressive disturbances in spermatogenesis were evident during serial testicular biopsies done in the course of experiments on these severely stressed male prisoners. In some cases, the arrest of spermatogenesis was so extreme that only the Sertoli cells and primordial spermatogonia were found in the tubules of the testes, which had been normal at the start of the experiment.

In one of our own patients an acute emotional shock caused a marked depression in spermatogenesis. The patient's semen was of borderline quality over several years, with sperm counts averaging 30 million per ml. and 40 per cent good motility with passable morphology. His wife had twice conceived and delivered a normal child. This man was asleep in the back seat of a car driven by his brother on a cross-country trip to a family reunion. There was an accident in which his brother was killed instantly but from which the patient emerged unharmed. When he was next seen by us 2 months after the accident, his sperm count had dropped to close to azoospermic levels, and it remained that way for 4 months before returning to the level at which it had been prior to the accident.

It is often difficult to ascribe an individual case of faulty human spermatogenesis to emotional factors because of the lack of well-controlled studies before and after exposure to the stress situation. However, such studies have been performed in animals with experiments designed to investigate the effects of repeated frustration and other types of stress situations such as overcrowding. Depression of spermatogenesis has been a well-documented effect,[49] and studies on such animals using radiolabeled spermatozoa have shown that sperm conduction time through the ductal system is markedly prolonged during situations of stress. Stress has also been shown to inhibit testicular monoamine oxidase (MAO) activity. Decreased monoamine oxidase levels could cause an increase in potentially damaging biogenic amines such as serotonin,[193] which in turn could have a sperm-depleting effect on the seminiferous tubules.[21, 100] This is believed to be due to a direct harmful effect of serotonin on spermatogenesis and not to a decrease in luteinizing-hormone release from the pituitary. Normal Leydig cell histology also verifies the fact that testosterone synthesis does not change.

Animal studies using paragylene (Parnate), an MAO inhibitor, have shown that there is a sloughing of immature cells into the lumina of the seminiferous tubules; the depletion of mature spermatozoa after long-term paragylene administration resembles the typical seminal stress pattern often noted in oligospermic infertility patients.[108]

The stress-related increase in serotonin levels noted with inhibited monoamine oxidase activity can in turn increase prostaglandin synthesis and activity[169] which has been shown to produce an increase in the force and rate of seminiferous tubular contractions.[40] Indeed, increased excretion levels of serotonin have been found in oligospermic and azoospermic men,[169] and it is postulated that hydralazine, a vasodilator, might prevent the harmful effect of serotonin.[21]

In relation to the stress-related psychogenic aspects of human infertility, mention should be made of the mistaken belief that it is common for couples to conceive *after* the *adoption of a child* as the resolution of an infertility problem. Although it has been shown statistically that adoption, resulting in the physical presence of a baby in the home of the infertile couple, does not increase the chances that conception will occur,[148, 161, 198] one does hear of occasional cases in which a child was conceived after adoption, and in these cases reduction of stress and anxiety in the marriage may be a factor.[1, 9] However, the pregnancy may have been due to unpublicized donor insemination, statistics of which are notoriously unreliable.

AGE

In general, age plays little or no role in sperm production in the group of patients in the 20- to 60-year age group who consult the doctor about infertility problems. (We know very little about the ejaculate content of young boys because of the difficulty in obtaining such specimens.) The aging process in the male gonad is not as marked or as uniform as it is in the female gonad. Hypospermatogenesis does occur in the aged and is probably related to the thickening of the basement membranes of the tubules,[41] but unless some disease is present, production of sperm does not cease abruptly at any time. We have several patients who have become fathers in their mid-sixties, and viable sperm can be found even in very elderly men. Although fertility is reduced, there are reliable reports of men becoming fathers at 80, or even 90 years of age.[153, 171] Live sperm have been found in the ejaculates of men in their nineties.[196]

DIABETES

The vascular changes induced by diabetes may accelerate the aging process. In addition, the diabetic patient may be heir to other problems affecting his fertility. Impotence occurs at an unusually high rate among diabetic men, and indeed may be the first symptom of this disease. The retrograde ejaculation of semen due to diabetic neuropathy has been frequently encountered. Further consideration of the management of problems of diabetic men desiring to have children is found in Chapter 10.

FREQUENCY OF COITUS

Although daily ejaculation may have no clinically significant effect on the sperm count of a man who normally has a high sperm concentration, such a practice can further reduce an already poor count.[51] Sexual relations every other day are generally preferable during the fertile period if the sperm count is borderline. As mentioned earlier, sperm motility can be depressed by prolonged continence.

Spermatozoa live within the ductus epididymis for a much longer time than they do in the female reproductive tract or *in vitro*. Sperm longevity in the epididymis has been observed to be as great as 30 to 70 days in the rat, rabbit, guinea pig, and bull, and several months in certain species of bats. Therefore, the ability of the spermatozoon to contribute to a viable embryo is lost before it loses its ability to fertilize eggs, and it loses its fertilizing capacity before it loses motility. These senescent changes are manifest in the spermatozoon by changes in the Feulgen reactivity response in the nucleus and by an increased eosinophilia. (The Feulgen reaction is a staining technique used to study the localization of DNA in the nucleus.)

After prolonged periods of abstinence from ejaculation, the ejaculate often contains a higher than normal proportion of dead and senescent spermatozoa, and it is possible that such spermatozoa could be a cause of embryonic death or fetal abnormality.[116]

RADIATION

The harmful effects of x-rays on the testes have been known ever since the report of Albers-Schönberg in 1903 describing azoospermia and infertility in guinea pigs and rabbits subsequent to irradiation.[2] It was shown in 1905 and again in 1907 that x-rays cause degeneration of the cells lining the seminal canals without diminishing sexual potency.[27, 143] Early in the investigation of the effects of x-rays on the testes, it became apparent that the cells of Leydig and Sertoli are relatively resistant to ionizing radiation. Germinal cells are sensitive and may disappear for prolonged periods after irradiation. However, the different types of germinal epithelial cells vary in radiosensitivity. Spermatids and spermatocytes are relatively resistant.[93] Spermatocytes are damaged by fairly high doses, but the effect is not evident until the irradiated primary spermatocytes undergo the first cell divisions in maturation. With relatively low doses of radioactivity significant damage is limited to the spermatogonia. The spermatogonial loss induces gradual depopulation of the seminiferous tubules as the progeny of the spermatogonia do not appear. This phenomenon is the so-called maturation depletion following irradiation.

There have been various suggestions to explain the loss of spermatogonia after irradiation: (1) direct destruction of these cells, (2) inhibition of spermatogonial mitosis, and (3) premature maturation of spermatogonia. In 1959 Oakberg demonstrated, by using the technique of enumerating the types of spermatogonia at the various stages of the cycle of the seminiferous epithelium, aided by better techniques for standardization of radiation doses delivered to the testicular tissue, that radiation caused direct destruction of the spermatogonia and that this was the most important and perhaps the only factor in the mechanism for spermatogonial depletion by irradiation.[131] Direct irradiation of mature ejaculated spermatozoa, in which the nuclei are in the resting state, usually has little or no effect on the motility, survival, morphology, or metabolism of sperm. Nevertheless, irradiated spermatozoa may be incapable of fertilizing or of inducing normal development of the ovum owing to damaged chromatin.[114]

The occurrence of detrimental mutants is predicted in three of every five children of men who have received a total of 225 or more rads of irradiation to their gonads during their prepubertal years.[72] In view of this fact, serious attempts should be made to weigh the need for diagnostic irradiation and especially therapeutic irradiation in boys.[82] After irradiation damage of the adult testes has occurred, years may be required for reconstruction of the germinal epithelium. This damage is apparently proportionate to the dosage received and probably causes azoospermia in men with poor spermatogenesis more quickly than in those with normal production of sperm. Radiation that causes considerable damage to the testes may be followed by recovery of fertility, as documented in a report in 1964.[111] In June 1958, a radiation accident occurred in one of the nuclear plants at Oak Ridge, Tennessee, and eight men were exposed to radioactive uranium. At least five of the men received sufficient total body radiation (236 to 365 rads) to produce symptoms of acute radiation syndrome, and they were found to be virtually sterile within 4 months after the accident. Their semen was examined at intervals and recovery of spermatogenesis was found to occur within 21 months of radiation exposure, although a reasonable level of fertility was not attained until 41 months after exposure.

Since the selective destruction of the sperm-forming elements in the testicles by x-rays and other forms of radiation is well documented, it follows that the testicles should at all times be guarded from unnecessary exposure to sources of radiation. Doctors, dentists, and x-ray technicians in particular should protect their gonads from exposure to x-rays. Had proper shielding been utilized in the 1950s by the shoe salesmen who used fluoroscopes to demonstrate correct fitting, fertility problems would not have occurred. Fortunately, such devices are now outlawed.

Potentially adverse effects on fertility are thought to occur in young men treated for a testicular tumor by *unilateral orchiectomy and radiation therapy*. The tumor dose for seminoma without demonstrable metastasis is up to 3000 rads within 19 to 25 days. For other histologic types of tumors without metastasis up to 5500 rads are applied within 33 to 52 days. The actual period of treatment depends on the quality of radiation and the patient's tolerance of the radiation. To deliver the tumor dose, a multiple fixed field technique must be used. In a patient with seminoma it is usually possible to give the dose by two directly opposed anterior and posterior fields. However, when the higher tumor dose (5000 or more rads) is needed, a multiple converging field technique is necessary.

Treatment for seminoma consists of high inguinal (or radical) orchiectomy with postoperative irradiation of the pathways of lymphatic drainage, at least to a level immediately above the renal pedicles. This technique is recommended for all adult patients in the absence of demonstrated widely disseminated disease. The remaining testis and scrotum are shielded during therapy. Whether the apparatus delivers 2 million electron volts or 400 or 250 kilovolts, doses of radiation to the shielded scrotal surface overlying the remaining testis, using current treatment techniques, approach 2 per cent of the surface doses of the pelvic fields, thus exposing the remaining testis to considerable radiation. The shield protecting the testis does not reduce this measured dose, indicating that the major source of radiation to the shielded testis is scattered primarily from the patient's body.[133]

In 1970, we reported on the restoration of spermatogenesis in seven men who had been rendered azoospermic after unilateral radical inguinal orchiectomy and postoperative radiation therapy for testicular tumors.[6] In five men, four of whom were known to have normal preoperative fertility levels, the semen quality fell to the level of azoospermia and was restored to normal levels within 3 to 4 years after therapy. Three of these patients subsequently fathered apparently normal children. The remaining two patients with seminoma who were known to have poor semen quality were subjected to similar therapy and rendered azoospermic. Four years later the semen of both had been restored to its former poor quality. Hence, one can infer that unilateral orchiectomy and radiation therapy need not be permanently damaging to male fertility if the patient has been cured of his malignant disease.

DRUGS AND CHEMICALS AFFECTING SPERMATOGENESIS

A number of drugs have a sterilizing action in men, either by affecting the several stages of spermatogenesis or by rendering the mature sperm incapable of fertilizing the egg. *Busulfan (Myleran),* used in the treatment of leukemia,[76, 77] has a destructive effect in the earliest stages of spermatogenesis, and *triethylenemelamine (TEM),* another alkylating agent, has been shown to produce temporary sterility in both early and late stages of spermatogenesis of rats.[22] Alkylating agents are radiomimetic — like radiation, these drugs selectively damage the germ cells.[172] In animal studies the drug effect appears to be dose-dependent.[178] At higher dosages, however, there is a strong possibility that azoospermia may be permanent. *Chlorambucil* used in the treatment of malignant lymphoma has caused azoospermia in therapeutic doses.[144] *Cyclophosphamide,* which is now used to treat rheumatoid arthritis as well as the nephrotic syndrome and glomerulonephritis, especially in children, causes a severe drop in spermatogenesis to the level of azoospermia and should be reserved for those patients in whom the consequences of either prolonged steroid treatment or the disease itself outweigh the risk of sterility.[43, 87]

Awareness of the side effects of chemotherapeutic agents should be increased, since in recent years the use of drug therapy for malignant diseases as well as for a variety of nonmalignant disorders has increased dramatically. Because these chemotherapeutic agents in lower species have been shown to be mutagenic, often producing a self-aborting conceptus,[12] there is much concern about the quality of sperm in men who experience return of spermatogenesis after chemotherapy. This is particularly true for *methotrexate,* which is currently in vogue for treating psoriasis.[39, 149] The original insight into the therapeutic efficiency of the antimetabolites against psoriasis arose from observations in leukemia patients who also had psoriasis. Methotrexate is an antimetabolite that interferes with folic acid metabolism in nucleic acid synthesis. It is an undesirable drug from the viewpoint of the physician dealing with fertility problems because it has the potential for producing chromosomal abnormalities in the germinal cells. Methotrexate has been used to sterilize house flies and screw-worm flies in insect control.[26]

Colchicine, used for centuries in the therapy of gout, has recently been shown to be beneficial in the prevention of attacks of Mediterranean fever. Merlin[118] reported that colchicine therapy caused azoospermia in a patient whose fertility was restored when the drug was discontinued. Harmful effects from high doses of colchicine on spermatogenesis in laboratory animals have also been documented.[14, 15, 138, 150] Colchicine is an agent used by geneticists to arrest meiosis in the spindle stage in chromosomal studies. Serreira and Buoniconti[170] found that because patients taking colchicine frequently have only 47 chromosomes in lymphocytic cultures, this drug might lead to a greater than normal risk of a trisomic offspring.

Bremner and Paulsen[20] studied seven normal males aged 20 to 25 years to determine whether colchicine had an effect on testicular function. They found that colchicine in therapeutic doses did not depress sperm counts in normal subjects and suggested that possibly in some gouty patients the testes are more susceptible to toxic effects from colchicine, although they studied one gouty patient who had normal sperm counts while on chronic colchicine therapy. They suggest that if infertility is a problem in a man who is on colchicine therapy, seminal fluid analysis and cessation of the drug should be considered. In patients with gout, it would be preferable to use allopurinal, which is not detrimental to spermatogenesis.

Dilantin (diphenylhydantoin), widely used in the therapy of epilepsy and other nervous system disorders, has been found to depress both FSH levels and spermatogenesis, with resultant severe oligoasthenospermia in 8 of 24 patients on chronic Dilantin therapy.[181] Five of these patients were studied intensively and compared to a group of controls. It was found that Dilantin therapy selectively depressed FSH without producing discernible abnormalities in LH, testosterone, estradiol, or prolactin, and was associated with severe oligospermia (sperm counts in the range of 1 to 5 million per ml.) and poor sperm motility.

Aspirin in large doses has been found to cause an inhibition of prostaglandin E and F concentration in seminal fluid and plasma.[33] In one report a deficiency of prostaglandins was found in the seminal fluid of 40 per cent of males with unexplained infertility.[28] A possible connection between high intake of aspirin and infertility must be considered in some men who receive large doses of aspirin for prolonged periods of time. The effect of aspirin on seminal fluid prostaglandins is probably the result of inhibition of the enzyme prostaglandin–synthetase. Inhibition of this enzyme in cows and sheep has been shown to produce similar effects.[80]

The transplacental hazard of *diethylstilbestrol* (DES) to the developing fetus was first brought to the attention of the medical community by Herbst and co-workers,[69a, 69b] who correlated vaginal adenocarcinoma in young women with DES given during their mothers' pregnancies. These reports of clear cell adenocarcinomas and the more frequent adenosis of the vagina and cervix have been confirmed by several groups.[17a, 60a, 177a]

The efficacy of DES for the protection of pregnancy was evaluated by Dieckmann[35a] in 1953 at the University of Chicago's Lying-in Hospital with a prospective, double blind, random study of 2000 consecutively registered pregnancies. In all, 840 pregnant women received DES, and 806 received placebos. The follow-up of the female offspring confirmed Herbst's findings, as reported by Bibbo *et al.,*[17a, 17b] and their follow-up of male offspring was the first to report anatomic abnormalities in the male genital tract and abnormal semen analyses in a small number of the males who have been studied to date. This study, which is currently in progress, has described the occurrence of small testes, solitary epididymal cysts (usually at the globus major), small penis, and areas of induration of the testicular capsule in a small but significant percentage of males who were exposed to DES *in utero.* Poor semen quality was found in a smaller sample population of this study.[56a]

Recent scientific evidence has shown that *marihuana* is not at all harmless.[84, 126] It contains unique substances, the "cannabinoids," which are soluble only in fat and are stored for weeks and months in body tissues, including the testicles, in the same manner as DDT. An individual using marihuana more than once a week (the time required for its elimination) cannot be drug-free, in contrast to the use of tobacco or alcohol. Marihuana (cannabis) can cause chromosomal anomalies that can lead to genetic damage.[126] Studies show that many of the cultured lymphocytes from marihuana users are also structurally abnormal: 30 per cent of these cells in metaphase contained only 5 to 30 chromosomes, whereas in nonusers only 7 per cent of these cells were abnormal. Similar findings have been reported in lung cultures exposed to marihuana smoke. These studies have led to speculation that marihuana products accumulating in testes (and ovaries) might also interfere with DNA metabolism of the germ cells. Such alterations of the gonads indicate that marihuana might have mutagenic effects. Cannabis may act on hormone regulators and produce impotence and temporary sterility. Kolodny *et al.*[83] recently reported sperm counts and testosterone levels that were low to the point of temporary infertility in the marihuana smoker; these low levels were probably related to retention of the drug in the testes. We strongly advise our patients against the use of marihuana. It is not a harmless substance.

The excessive use of *alcohol* may contribute to liver damage which may in turn lead to failure to detoxify estrogen in the male, with a resultant depression of sperm production. Alcohol ingested and then partially excreted in the seminal fluid has been shown to decrease fertility in humans,[4] but this effect has been poorly documented.

In addition to its many deleterious physiologic effects,[188] heavy *tobacco* smoking may cause some depression of sperm production, although no significant well-controlled experimental studies of this effect have been reported in the literature.

A study was carried out in Switzerland on 150 workmen who had long-term exposure to *lead* while working in a storage battery factory.[89] Anlaysis of the semen of lead-poisoned workers showed low sperm counts, poor sperm motility, and abnormal forms in the ejaculates. An increased number of sperm with duplicate, tapering, or amorphous heads was present, and there were complaints of decreased libido and difficulties of erection and ejaculation. These data indicate that long-term exposure to lead has an adverse effect on fertility. Suggestions for the protection of fertility in workmen exposed to lead include clinical and toxicologic checkups, temporary interruption of exposure and chelate therapy in men showing moderately increased lead absorption or lead poisoning, and maintenance of lead concentrations that do not exceed the minimum permissible levels at the working sites.

Arsenic may replace phosphorus in the synthesis of DNA.[199] Since *zinc* ions are toxic to sperm, an increase in the zinc levels in the seminal fluid may cause coiling of sperm tails *in vitro*, which can be reversed by the addition of albumin.[96, 151] In studies of the split ejaculate it was found that addition of seminal fluid from the first (prostatic) fraction improved the motility of sperm from the second (seminal vesicular) fraction, and it has been inferred that the albumin in the first fraction exerts a protective effect due to the binding of free zinc ions.[78, 97] On the other hand, no significant differences in such electrolytes as *sodium, potassium, calcium,* or *magne-*

sium ions have been found in the seminal plasma content of normal and abnormal ejaculates, and no relationship has been found between changes in these electrolyte concentrations in the spermatozoal environment and poor sperm motility.[25]

NUTRITION

Good nutrition certainly plays a helpful role in the continuous production of sperm cells. A diet well balanced in proteins, fats, carbohydrates, vitamins, and minerals is essential. Numerous investigations have shown the influence of nutritional status on the normal development and function of male gonads.[18, 92] Generalizations are difficult in view of the lack of standardization of experimental diets, the complex nature of the constituents of many diets, and also our meager knowledge of the interactions that occur in simple and multiple deficiencies. In many cases, it is not known whether there is a direct effect on the germinal epithelium or whether it is mediated through some systemic pathway.

Men with an otherwise unexplained decline in spermatogenesis may have been on severe "crash" diets for rapid weight loss; their semen quality returns to its previous level when their diet returns to normal. This phenomenon may be analogous to that in women with hypothalamic hypogonadotropic amenorrhea associated with poor nutrition.

Several amino acids have been detected in human semen. They have been thought to play a role in spermatozoal activity.[54] Among invertebrates the addition of any one of a number of amino acids and peptides to spermatozoa extends their duration of motility.[152] Several amino acids have been used to treat cases of oligospermia and asthenospermia with varying degrees of success. Of the amino acids utilized for this purpose, *arginine* has received the most attention, and there have been several reports of encouraging results.[17, 74, 162, 184] However, many of the reports are anecdotal, the dosages and follow-up varied, and the clinical response was unpredictable. Mroueh[124] evaluated the effect of arginine in oligospermia and correlated any improvement with the specific histologic appearance of the testis biopsy in 28 men. He found no definite improvement in semen quality regardless of pathology in patients given 2 gm. of arginine hydrochloride daily for 10 weeks. Our own clinical experience with arginine therapy (see Chapter 9) has also been disappointing.

There is no question that *vitamin E* deficiency in the rat results in specific and irreversible damage to the testes. Tubular damage may proceed to the point where only Sertoli cells remain, yet the interstitial cells are not affected.[117] Little or no effect from an absence of vitamin E has been noted in humans, however.[101] Severe *vitamin A* deficiency in humans produces a progressive loss of germinal cells, starting with the most mature, but affects spermatogonia and spermatocytes relatively little. Testis damage induced by vitamin A deficiency can be reversed, but vitamin A therapy in man for oligospermia not due to lack of the vitamin has no effect.[70] *Vitamin B–complex* deficiencies have been demonstrated to cause regressive changes in the male accessory organs of rats that can be reversed by the administration of testicular hormone or anterior pituitary extracts.[122] It has been concluded that the primary lesion due to B–complex deficiency is located in the pituitary gland and that because of diminished hypophyseal activity, the testes receive insufficient gonadotropic stimulation. This results in too little male sex hormone to support the normal functioning of the accessory glands, a state called "pseudohypophysectomy."[59]

Vitamin C (ascorbic acid) may have a therapeutic role in the prevention of sperm agglutination because it is a reducing agent. There is an antiagglutinin present in semen that exists in both an oxidized and a reduced state but is active only when it is in the chemically reduced state. When reduction fails to take place, relatively poor antiagglutinin activity is noted. The reduced form of antiagglutinin is attached to the surface of the spermatozoon and loses its ability to become fixed to the cell surface when oxidized.[95] The therapeutic management of these patients is based on the oral administration of ascorbic acid,[88] a naturally occurring, potent reducing agent found in semen. Ascorbic acid, given in doses of 500 mg. four times daily, has been found to be most effective. A normal semen picture and sperm motility reappear in many cases when the sperm agglutination is not caused by immunologic factors.

INFECTIONS

Mumps. With regard to fertility, the most clinically significant testicular infection is postpubertal mumps orchitis. Although mumps before puberty usually does not cause orchitis, there is a relatively high incidence of testicular involvement on one or both sides when the virus infection occurs after puberty. The onset of orchitis is usually 4 to 6 days after the appearance of the parotitis, but it may occur without parotid involvement. In about 70 per cent of cases, the orchitis is unilateral, with some degree of atrophy of the involved testis in half of the cases in which there has been testicular enlargement. If the atrophy is bilateral, sterility will result. We have treated several patients who had severe bilateral mumps orchitis with no ensuing atrophy; in these men there was only a temporary severe depression of spermatogenesis and full recovery occurred within 6 to 10 months. One such patient had six children prior to his attack of bilateral mumps orchitis and was actually hoping that he would be rendered sterile, but he had an excellent semen analysis 8 months later, and child number seven was born 21 months after his infection. Anti-inflammatory corticoids offer the best adjuvant therapy for mumps orchitis.

Tuberculosis. Tuberculosis does not ordinarily involve the testes, but it can occasionally produce destructive granuloma with necrosis, abscess formation, and tubular atrophy. Extratesticular involvement with obstruction of the epididymis and vas deferens is more common. Epididymal involvement in tuberculosis usually follows a prostatic or seminal vesicle lesion.[87] Nine cases of transmission of genital tuberculosis to the wife from a husband with untreated tuberculosis of the epididymis through the semen have been reported in the American and European literature.[90] Azoospermia results from the bilateral obstruction of the vas and epididymis by tuberculosis. Restoration of the patency of the vas, shown by the reappearance of sperm in the semen, has been reported; apparently recanalization around the cold abscess occurred. It is recommended that the removal of a tuberculous epididymis be avoided if possible, since chemotherapy will usually suffice. If the disease is arrested, an occlusion may occasionally be overcome by epididymovasostomy, but because of the usual extensive scarring of the ductal system the prognosis is poor.

Gonorrhea. Gonorrhea not only involves severe inflammatory changes in the urethra and prostate but can also cause severe epididymitis. Due to adequate antibiotic therapy, the postinflammatory obstructive lesions of untreated gonorrhea which produce ductal blockage at the tail of the epididymis are fortunately uncommon. These lesions occasionally still cause obstructive azoospermia. They may be a major cause of infertility in those areas of the world where gonorrhea is not promptly and adequately treated.

Acute Nonspecific Epididymitis. Unsatisfactory resolution of acute nonspecific epididymitis may also result in ductal blockage on the involved side; if bilateral, it may result in sterility that requires bypass surgery for management. Although the clinical aspects of the infection may seem to involve only the epididymis, there is frequently a concomitant inflammatory involvement of the testis, with reduction in spermatogenesis and possible subsequent atrophy of the germinal epithelium.[130] Prompt and intensive antibiotic therapy is necessary during the acute phase of epididymitis to prevent obstruction and damage to the testicular germinal cells.

Prostatitis. Acute prostatitis may produce impotence. Although there are no conclusive reports of a correlation between prostatitis and infertility, the presence of *Escherichia coli* and related organisms is known to cause sperm agglutination in the infected ejaculum and to depress sperm motility *in vitro*.[141, 187] Prostatitis should be treated and cleared up if possible. If the infection is treated, it is best to avoid the use of nitrofurantoin (Furadantin) because of its detrimental effects on spermatogenesis.

T-Mycoplasma Infection. There has been speculation that infection with the T (for tiny) forms of mycoplasma may be associated with infertility in couples. The first mycoplasmas to be isolated from a human in 1937 came from a Bartholin's abscess.[36] Since then much interest has been centered on the relationhsip between mycoplasmas found in the genitourinary tract and disease. Although T-mycoplasmas are commonly found in the genitourinary tracts of adults, there is still no clear evidence that these organisms play a pathogenic role.[102, 103] However, T-mycoplasmas have been shown to occur more frequently in the ejaculates and cervical secretions of couples with unexplained infertility than in fertile couples,[57, 58, 62] and pregnancies were achieved in about 30 per cent of infertile couples after eradication of the T-mycoplasmas by antibiotics.[71] Fowlkes *et al.*[45] studied the morphology of T-mycoplasmas in cultures and in semen from men with infertile marriages. Using scanning electron microscopy, they observed a physical association between the microorganism and spermatozoa which may contribute to decreased motility of spermatozoa in semen. In further studies[46] they suggested that the mycoplasma organisms may adhere to the midpiece of the spermatozoa, causing some impediment to normal motile activity. Although these data support the hypothesis that T-mycoplasmas may play a role in human infertility, the need for further investigation is shown by contrary findings by Mardh and Westrom,[115] who isolated T-mycoplasmas more frequently from pregnant (68 per cent) than from nonpregnant women (46 per cent), and by Taylor-Robinson and Manchee,[185] who reported a 25 per cent pregnancy rate in a group of previously infertile women carrying mycoplasma. Patton and Taymor[134] found no relationship between the quality of the postcoital test and the presence of mycoplasma. Also, it has been noted that bovine semen samples have a high fertilizing capacity despite the fact that practically all samples contain T-mycoplasmas.[185] Mycoplasma organisms, especially T-mycoplasmas, are difficult to culture, and few clinical laboratories have the necessary facilities. Consequently, the evaluation of T-mycoplasma infections still requires research.

It is clear that T-mycoplasmas do not affect sperm count and consequently are not a cause of oligospermia. A recent prospective study has failed to demonstrate either a significant increase in T-mycoplasma infections in barren couples or a significant effect of T-mycoplasmas on primary infertility.[35] As more and more articles are published, T-mycoplasma as a possible agent in infertility seems less and less likely, and unless there is further confirmation of the beneficial effects of tetracycline in cases in which the infection is suspect, the empirical use of this drug should be avoided.

Smallpox. Azoospermia has been found in a strikingly high percentage of men who have had smallpox. Eighty per cent have obstructive lesions in the epididymis.[137] In India, smallpox infection is the single most important and most frequently encountered causative factor which produces obstructive azoospermia in man.

Leprosy (Hansen's Disease). Lepromatous leprosy produces granulomatous lesions with obstructive azoospermia, which accounts for the high incidence of infertility in lepromatous males.[135] It has been suggested that the extinction of leprosy in France during the 17th century was a consequence of the law obliging leprous persons to marry among themselves.[86]

PARAPLEGIA

In a review of the physiology of the testes, Hotchkiss[72] notes that severe degeneration of the seminiferous tubules results from denervation of the lumbar spinal nerves that probably pass through the sympathetic trunk, including the third, fourth, fifth, and sixth lumbar ganglia. The pain and thermoregulatory centers may reside at about the level of T10 to T12.[179, 183] The atrophy of the germinal epithelium may be due to paralysis of the blood vessels, thereby causing alterations of testicular temperature incompatible with spermatogenesis.[123] Hypertrophy of the Leydig cells has been noted as a parallel development to spermatogenic failure, and increased amounts of androgens and estrogens appear in the urine of some paraplegic men. It may be inferred that one consequence of spermatogenic failure is the lack of a check on the pituitary gland, which results in increased elaboration of LH and thereby stimulates the steroid-producing cells.

In paraplegic patients who desire to retain their fertility potential, consideration should be given to freeze-preservation of semen obtained as early as possible after the injury.

CHRONIC RENAL FAILURE, DIALYSIS, AND RENAL TRANSPLANTATION

Endocrine dysfunction, including impotence, loss of libido, testicular atrophy, alterations in testicular histology, and gynecomastia, has been reported in patients with chronic renal failure. Chronic uremia results in low levels of circulating testosterone, possibly due to an impaired pituitary-Leydig cell function. Patients with uremia maintained on chronic hemodialysis showed severe oligospermia with poor sperm motility; severe germinal-cell arrest at the primary spermatocyte stage was evident on biopsy of testes. Libido improves in some patients on chronic dialysis, although spermatogenesis often remains impaired.[189] Following transplantation, libido, potency, and ejaculatory reflexes may improve dramatically soon after the transplanted kidney resumes normal function.[159] These characteristics may again regress during acute or chronic rejection. In the Cleveland Clinic series, Stewart[180] reported 10 normal children fathered by patients who had undergone successful renal homotransplantation. However, the great majority of patients on immunosuppressive therapy following transplantation remained significantly oligospermic, probably as a result of the relatively high doses of steroids and azathioprine given to them. Other factors, such as local radiation of the graft (for rejection crisis) and extensive surgery during the transplant procedure, may have adversely affected the fertility potential. Restoration of ovulatory function and subsequent motherhood in women undergoing renal transplantation have also been reported. Experience to date indicates, that, although fertility potential is reduced in both men and women following renal transplantation, parenthood is distinctly possible, and contraceptive measures should always be advised unless the couple actively desire more children.

ALLERGIC REACTIONS

An acute allergic reaction may produce a profound temporary disruption of spermatogenesis. There is a well-documented case of temporary sterility following a violent reaction to Merthiolate.[108] Severe reactions to penicillin have also been known to produce temporary sterility in previously fertile men.

There are only two reports actually documenting a typical allergic response of the wife to her husband's ejaculate.[61, 94] In each of these cases the wife developed a severe and reproducible allergic reaction within a few minutes after intercourse, characterized by itchy swollen eyes, nasal congestion, sneezing, perivaginal swelling and itching, diffuse urticaria, and laryngeal edema. This reaction did not occur when a condom was used or when coitus interruptus was employed during intercourse, but the severe allergic episode occurred each time these preventive measures were not employed successfully. This allergic syndrome is fortunately very uncommon.

IMMUNOLOGIC FACTORS AND INFERTILITY

In recent years it has become increasingly apparent that immunologic factors in both men and women can play a role in the process of reproduction.[112, 173] Inherent in the immunologic processes is the ability of a host to recognize foreign antigens. Since the various parts of the male reproductive system do not attain functional maturity until puberty, and since most of the components are not only unique but are also released outside the body, the developing individual has no opportunity to recognize these components as self-antigen. Therefore, it is not surprising that any antigen that is not present during the time the body is developing tolerance to self-antigens can at a later time evoke an immunologic response upon exposure. The various parts of the germinal epithelium develop within the blood–testis barrier, preventing any passage of serum proteins into the seminiferous tubules.[79]

Although the antigenicity of sperm has been known for more than 75 years,[119] the initial findings of an autoimmune phenomenon occurring in men must be credited to Wilson[200, 201] and Rümke.[154] Wilson demonstrated that, in three infertile human males, two with normal sperm counts and the third with oligospermia, sperm agglutinating antibodies were present in the seminal plasma and in the blood sera. In two of these cases, in which donor insemination was attempted, conception promptly occurred. Rümke[154] found the serum of two oligospermic males capable of agglutinating the sperm of normal men, and believed the occurrence might have resulted from some autoimmunization process. It should be noted that Rümke used the Kibrick sperm agglutinating method[81] for his studies. His initial observations led to an investigation of the possible presence of sperm antibodies (agglutinins) in the blood sera of both normal sterile men.[157] None of the fertile men demonstrated significant titers of agglutinins for human sperm, whereas approximately 3 per cent of the childless males showed significant titers. The majority of the reacting sera produce tail-to-tail agglutination, but others produced head-to-head clumping and mixtures of both types. Rümke also studied the occurrence of occlusions or other obstructions in sperm ducts of a large number of azoospermic males. A positive correlation was found between obstruction and the presence of sperm agglutinins in the serum. It was suggested that this might serve as a basis for autoimmunization, which might cause sperm agglutination in the ejaculate of males in whom obstruction occurred only on one side or was due to an inflammation when the occlusion was temporary.

Tyler and Bishop[192] pointed out that there were other possible explanations for autoimmunization. For example, the antibodies might have been formed in response to some related antigen from other tissues or from outside the body, or they may have resulted from some derangement of a normal system of complementary substances leading to complement-fixation phenomenon. Rümke in 1974[156] demonstrated conclusively that repeated injections of either sperm or testicular homogenates without Freund's complete adjuvant would lead to the development of circulating antibodies but would not induce testicular damage of the type demonstrated by Mancini et al. when they injected testicular material with Freund's complete adjuvant.[113] This allergic orchitis was experimentally induced by Mancini et al. in the guinea pig, rat, rhesus monkey, and man. Cytologically the lesion consists of progressive cytolysis of the germinal epithelium but does not appear to affect the Sertoli or Leydig cell populations. While this experimental aspermatogenesis may serve as a theoretical model for male infertility, there is no evidence that such a phenomenon appears spontaneously despite various reports of circulating antibodies and sperm agglutinins in infertile males.[155, 157]

Two different groups of antigens have been reported. One group is common to the testis, epididymis, and spermatozoa, and the other is present in the adnexal glands and their fluid. In allergic orchitis, the histologic lesion appears in 1 to 8 weeks and is reversible after 24 weeks. By using immunofluorescent microscopy, the antibody appears to be localized in the acrosomal region of both spermatozoa and spermatids. No strict correlation has been shown to exist between the severity of the gonadal lesion and the titer of the circulating antibody. Cell-bound antibodies involved with delayed hypersensitivity, may be more important, as has been suggested in recent studies of lymphocyte transformation using seminal plasma from infertile men.[125]

Rümke and Hellinga conjectured in 1959 that autoantibodies to sperm may form in certain men because of an acquired obstruction in some part of the ductal system and that this blockage, by causing back pressure and extravasation of sperm into the interstitial tissue, stimulates antibody formation.[157] Phadke and Padukone[136] also suggested this in 1964 when they reported that sperm-agglutinating antibodies were found in the sera from 5 (20 per cent) of 25 men with acquired obstruction of the ductal system and from 8 (32 per cent) of 25 men who had been sterilized by vasoligation. The occurrence of sperm-agglutinating antibodies as an immunologic consequence of vasectomy was confirmed by Rümke[155] in 1968 and by Zappi et al.[203] in 1970. In 1970 Ansbacher[10] initiated a long-term prospective study of sperm antibodies in vasectomized men and reported that, of the sera from 106 men tested before vasectomy, only one demonstrated an agglutinating antibody (titer 1:4). Two years after vasectomy 62 per cent had circulating sperm agglutinins, as demonstrated by the macroscopic gelatin sperm-agglutination test (SPAT) of Kibrick et al. (see Chapter 5 for further details of this test).[81] Antibodies against the sperm were demonstrated in the sera within 1 week after bilateral vasoligation. Similar findings have been reported by Shulman et al.[175] and Coombs et al.[34]

Operations designed to reverse vasectomy have been reported to result in reappearance of sperm in the ejaculate of up to 90 per cent of the patients, but these patients produced few pregnancies.[73] This low fertility rate after successful reanastomosis of the ligated vas may be attributable, at least in part, to the postvasectomy development of autoantibodies.

One small group of sterile men—those with congenital bilateral absense of the vasa—has recently been receiving more attention from urologists, reproductive biologists, and geneticists. These men are born with normally functioning testicles but have a "natural" vasectomy before birth. They are sterile because their sperm cannot escape from the globus major of the epididymis where, at exploration, these sperm can usually be found in large numbers.[8] This is not as small a group of men as was previously believed. Indeed, congenital bilateral absence of the vas deferens was found to be the cause of sterility in 2 per cent of over 5000 infertile patients examined in our urologic practice.[7] Because of the recent emphasis on immunologic aspects of infertility,[11] we set out to test for circulating sperm agglutinins in our patients with congenital bilateral absence of the vasa deferentia; all were azoospermic patients who had never had sperm cells in their ejaculates. Significantly high titers (1:32 to 1:4096) of sperm-agglutinating antibodies were found in 18 (62.1 per cent) of the 29 men (Table 4–1). The test was positive with low titers (1:16 or less) in five (17.2 per cent) of the men, and it was negative in six (20.7 per cent) of the men (Table 4–1).[7]

Whether sterilization was by elective vasectomy or by an embryologic

Table 4-1 TITERS OF CIRCULATING SPERM-AGGLUTINATING
ANTIBODIES IN 29 PATIENTS WITH AZOOSPERMIA
DUE TO CONGENITAL BILATERAL ABSENCE OF
THE VASA DEFERENTIA*

TITER[a]	NO. OF PATIENTS	% OF PATIENTS
0	6	20.7
1:4	2	
1:8	1	17.2
1:16	2	
1:32	1	
1:64	2	
1:128	2	
		62.1
1:256	7	
1:512	4	
≥1:1024	2	

*From Amelar, R. D., Dubin, L., and Schoenfeld, C.: Circulating sperm-agglu-
tinating antibodies in azoospermic men with congenital bilateral absence of the vasa
deferentia. Fertil. Steril., 26:228–231, 1975.
[a]Measured with Shulman's modification[174] of the macroscopic gelatin sperm-
agglutination test of Kibrick et al.[81]

developmental anomaly resulting in congenital bilateral absence of the vasa
deferentia, approximately 60 per cent of the patients had high titers of
sperm-agglutinating antibodies circulating in their sera. This coincidence
raises the question of whether development of sperm-agglutinating antibodies after vasectomy is caused by the particular surgical technique used or
simply by obstruction of the epididymis. Experimental procedures that
have been devised for the creation of artificial spermatoceles in patients
with congenital bilateral absence of the vasa[32, 63, 163–165] are prone to failure.
Some of the failures may be due to antibody interference.

We are still not entirely certain about the relationship of demonstrable
circulating sperm-agglutinating antibodies to subsequent fertility. For instance, Rümke and Hellinga[157] found in a study of 416 fertile men that
circulating sperm agglutinins occurred in four men but never in titers higher
than 1:16. Most recently, Rümke et al.[158] provided data from a long-term
study of the fertility status of 254 men who had been unable to father
children and who had sperm-agglutination titers ranging from 1:4 to greater
than 1:1024. The titers were detected with the Kibrick macroscopic sperm-
agglutination test. Of these, 36 had subsequently become fertile in the
years following serum testing. An inverse relationship between the serum
sperm-agglutination titer and the probability of becoming fertile was found
for these normospermic men. It is possible that serum titers of up to 1:16

have no clinical significance but above this ratio the significance increases markedly; only 7 of 91 normospermic men who had titers of 1:256 or higher eventually became fathers. The greatest decrease in probability of becoming fertile occurred in men with titers of between 1:16 and 1:32.

Isojima and his co-workers developed another immunologic test, which utilizes a sperm immobilization phenomenon first observed in the sera of women with unexplained infertility.[75] In their initial report 12 per cent of the women in the group with unexplained infertility demonstrated a complement dependent sperm-immobilizing antibody. This antibody has also been reported to occur in the male, especially after vasectomy.[10] In 30 per cent of vasectomized men this immobilizing antibody was present up to 1 year after vasectomy but declined in incidence to 9.5 per cent after 18 months; after 24 months a significant decline in titer and incidence was evident.

Still another means of testing for circulating sperm-agglutinating antibodies in both men and women, is the Franklin-Dukes microscopic method.[47, 48] In their report, 43 couples, all of whom were attempting to achieve a pregnancy for at least 2 years, demonstrated normal results from pelvic examination, Rubin test, hysterosalpingogram, endometrial biopsy, and a normal semen specimen from the husband. When the husband's sperm was mixed with the wife's serum and incubated for 4 hours at $37°$ C., 30 out of 43 (72.1 per cent) showed evidence of antispermatozoal antibody activity against the husband's sperm. This was in contrast to a group of couples with normal fertility in which only 2 of 35 couples demonstrated this phenomenon. When 13 husbands whose wives had the circulating antibody in their serum used condoms during intercourse or abstained for periods of 60 days to 6 months, the antibody titers declined markedly in all the women and were nondetectable in 10. These 10 women were instructed to resume unrestricted intercourse, carefully timed to coincide with ovulation, and nine were reported to have become pregnant.[48] The Franklin-Dukes (FD) test became a very popular method of searching for sperm-agglutinating antibodies until Boettcher and co-workers demonstrated that it did not measure immunoglobulins of the IgG or IgM type that were suspected to cause primary infertility, and that the FD test measured a beta-lipoprotein.[23, 24] In 1973 it was reported that the pregnancy rate among women with either primary or secondary infertility and a positive FD test was the same as that for a group of women with a primary or secondary infertility and a negative FD test.[132]

Transvaginal immunization is an interesting concept.[16] Immunoglobulins have been demonstrated in the female reproductive tract.[191] Human semen contains at least 16 antigens; spermatozoa have seven, four of which are identical with those of the seminal plasma.[142] It appears likely that sperm acquire antigens during their transit through the ductal system,[67] since these "coating" antibodies are present in seminal plasma in which no sperm are present. It would seem that when confronted with a case of unexplained infertility in which neither the husband nor the wife has demonstrable cause for infertility, the Kibrick test[81] for sperm-agglutinating antibodies and the Isojima test[75] for sperm-immobilizing antibodies should be performed on the sera of the couple. The reader is referred to Chapter 5 for complete information on the performance and interpretation of these tests. The infertile couple in whom an antispermatozoal antibody is demonstrated in the wife's serum should be advised to use a condom during intercourse for 60 days to 6 months, with monthly determinations of the antibody titer. When the antibody titer reaches its lowest point the probability of conception will be enhanced if normal coitus is resumed at the time of ovulation.

ANTIFERTILITY AGENTS

There has been a search for a substance which when fed or injected into men will arrest the process of sperm development in the testes. Using one line of approach, animals have been raised on unbalanced diets, which after a time cause an arrest in spermatogenesis. For example, it was found that when male rats were fed a diet supplement of 10 per cent or more of *erucic acid,* the fatty acid that is the major constituent of rapeseed oil, progressive reduction of spermatogenesis set in, and the animals became sterile after a few months.[65] It is probable that erucic acid acts by interfering with the metabolism of the essential fatty acids.

Certain drugs that were first found to be effective amoebicides were later discovered to be toxic to the testes in both animals and human beings. In 1960, it was found that *bis(dichloroacetyl)diamine,* a compound chemically related to chloramphenicol (Chloromycetin), suppressed spermatogenesis in 29 volunteer prisoners in a state penitentiary.[68] In 1961 this drug caused complete inhibition of spermatogenesis in a group of 60 volunteers in another state prison, and the profound effects were found to be completely reversible within several months.[107] Hopes that this might be the sought-for "birth-control pill" for men were dashed when it was found that men taking this drug became severely ill if they drank alcoholic beverages. Nevertheless, this study has led to further work, toward developing a pill which can temporarily produce male sterility with no unwanted side effects. Currently, experimentation is being carried out to combine bis (dichloroacetyl) diamine chemically with a steroid to produce an antifertility agent that has no antiabuse effects.

Testosterone, a sex hormone, has long been known to be an inhibitor of spermatogenesis, its effect being mediated by the pituitary and the suppression of gonadotropin secretion, with a consequent lowering of the high local concentration of testosterone within the testes.[69] Walsh and Swerdloff investigated the mechanism by which treatment with testosterone enanthate in either low or high dosages produced azoospermia in adult male rats.[197] They observed that low doses of testosterone enanthate

(0.3 mg. three times weekly for 6 weeks) decreased testis weight, produced atrophy of the germinal epithelium, and suppressed serum LH but not FSH. On the other hand, high doses (3.0 or 30.0 mg. three times weekly for 6 weeks) affected neither testis weight nor histology of the germinal epithelium and suppressed *both* LH and FSH. They concluded that testosterone induces germinal atrophy by suppressing serum LH concentrations and subsequent androgen production by the Leydig cells, thereby decreasing the normally high intratesticular levels of androgen that are necessary for maintenance of germinal epithelium. When these high concentrations of androgen are restored by injections of pharmacologic doses of testosterone, no disturbance of the germinal epithelium occurs despite suppression of both LH and FSH.

Another steroid, medroxyprogesterone acetate *(Depo-provera)*, has been found to cause a severe depression in both sperm count and motility after a single injection, probably by directly affecting the testes.[195]

Danazol affects spermatogenesis by its pituitary gonadotropin-inhibiting activity.[37, 60] It is orally active and is devoid of estrogen or progestational activity.[139] Recent research suggests that oral administration of this drug, in combination with testosterone to counteract its libido-reducing properties, may be an effective future method of suppressing fertility.[176]

Cyproterone acetate can cause a marked reduction in spermatogenesis, but it has no usefulness as an antifertility drug because it causes a marked inhibition of libido.[177]

Nitrofurantoin used clinically to combat urinary infections has been demonstrated to cause depression in spermatogenesis by interfering with carbohydrate metabolism in the germinal epithelium. It produces an arrest at the primary spermatocyte stage[127] and is known to cause temporary sterility in man. It seems apparent from the literature that the depression of spermatogenesis is related to dose.[128] The harmful effects of nitrofurantoin upon spermatogenesis[38, 140] are now so evident that this drug should not be used by the urologist to treat infections in men who have infertility problems. Indeed, the nitrofurans have been found to have sperm-immobilizing action and have been used to flush the vas during vasectomy to hasten the disappearance of spermatozoa from the ejaculate.[3]

In 1962, antidepressant drugs that are also *monoamine oxidase (MAO) inhibitors* (Nardil, Parnate, Niamid, Marplan) were noted, in a preliminary report by the Rockland State Hospital group,[19] to produce transient increase in the sperm count. However, the increase was followed by a profound drop to almost azoospermic levels with high numbers of abnormal cells. These drugs have undesirable side effects such as orthostatic hypotension that make them impractical for use in inducing infertility. Subsequent studies have demonstrated that testicular damage is produced by the MAO inhibitors, probably because of the secondary increase in serotonin levels, which have a sperm-depleting effect on the seminiferous tubules.[21, 100, 109]

REFERENCES

1. Abse, D. W.: Psychiatric aspects of male infertility. Fertil. Steril., *17*:133, 1966.
2. Albers-Schönberg: Über eine bisher unbekannte Wirkung der Rontgenstrahlen auf den Organisms der Tiere. Munch. Med. Wochenschr., *50*:1859, 1903.
3. Albert, P. S., Salerno, R. G., Kapoor, S. N., and Davis, J. E.: The nitrofurans as sperm-immobilizing agents, their tissue toxicity and their clinical applications in vasectomy. Fertil. Steril., *26*:485, 1975.
4. Albescú, J. Z., Bergadá, C., and Cullen, M.: Male fertility in patients treated for cryptorchidism before puberty. Fertil. Steril., *22*:829, 1971.
5. Amelar, R. D.: Infertility in Men: Diagnosis and Treatment. Philadelphia, F. A. Davis Co., 1966.
6. Amelar, R. D., Dubin, L., and Hotchkiss, R. S.: Restoration of fertility following unilateral orchiectomy and radiation therapy for testicular tumors. J. Urol., *106*:714, 1971.
7. Amelar, R. D., Dubin, L., and Schoenfeld, C.: Circulating sperm-agglutinating antibodies in azoospermic men with congenital bilateral absence of the vasa deferentia. Fertil. Steril., *26*:228, 1975.
8. Amelar, R. D., and Hotchkiss, R. S.: Congenital aplasia of the epididymides and vasa deferentia: effects on semen. Fertil. Steril., *14*:44, 1963.
9. Andrews, R. G.: Adoption and the resolution of infertility. Fertil. Steril., *21*:73, 1970.
10. Ansbacher, R.: Vasectomy: sperm antibodies. Fertil. Steril., *24*:788, 1973.
11. Ansbacher, R., Yeung, K. K., and Behrman, S. J.: Clinical significance of sperm antibodies in infertile couples. Fertil. Steril., *24*:305, 1973.
12. Auerbach, C.: Mutagenic effects of alkylating agents. Ann. N.Y. Acad. Sci., *68*:731, 1958.
13. Badenoch, A. W.: Descent of the testis in relation to temperature. Brit. Med. J., *2*:601, 1945.
14. Barsoum, H.: The effect of colchicine on the spermatogenesis of rabbits. J. Pharmacol., *115*:319, 1955.
15. Beatty, R. A., and Rowson, L. E. A.: Note on motility and fertility of colchicine-treated bull and rabbit sperm. J. Agricul. Sci., *45*:254, 1954.
16. Behrman, S. J., and Otani, Y.: Transvaginal immunization of the guinea pig with homologous testis and epididymal sperm. Int. J. Fertil., *8*:829, 1963.
17. Bernard, I.: Treatment of oligoastheno-spermia with arginine. *In* Westin, B. and Wiqvist, N. (eds.): Proceedings of the Fifth World Congress on Fertility and Sterility, Stockholm June 16–22, 1966. Amsterdam, Excerpta Medica Foundation, 1967, p. 898.
17a. Bibbo, M., Al-Naqeeb, M., Baccarini, I., Gill, W. B. *et al.*: Cytologic findings in female and male offspring of DES-treated mothers. Acta Cytol., *19*:568, 1975.
17b. Bibbo, M., Al-Naqeeb, M., Baccarini, I., Gill, W. B. *et al.*: Follow-up study of male and female offspring of DES-treated mothers. A preliminary report. J. Reprod. Med., *15*:29, 1975.
18. Bishop, M. W. H., and Walton, A.: Spermatogenesis and the structure of mammalian spermatozoa. *In* Parkes, A. S. (ed.): Marshalls' Physiology of Reproduction. 3rd ed. London, Longmans, Green and Co., Ltd., 1960, p. 88.
19. Blair, J. H., Simpson, G. M., and Kline, N. S.: Monoamine oxidase inhibitor and sperm production (Letter to the editor). J.A.M.A., *181*:172, 1962.
20. Bremner, W. J., and Paulsen, C. A.: Colchicine and testicular function in man. N. Engl. J. Med., *294*:1384, 1976.
21. Boccabella, A. V., Salgado, E. D., and Algar, E. A.: Testicular function and histology following serotonin administration. Endocrinology, *71*:827, 1962.
22. Bock, M., and Jackson, H.: The action of triethylinemelamine on the fertility of male rats. Brit. J. Pharmacol., *12*:1, 1957.
23. Boettcher, B., and Kay, D. J.: Fractionation of a human sperm-agglutinating serum. Nature, *223*:737, 1969.
24. Boettcher, B., Kay, D. J., Rümke, P., and Wright, L. E.: Human sera containing immunoglobulin and nonimmunoglobulin spermagglutinins. Biol. Reprod., *5*:236, 1971.
25. Bondani, A., Aspeita, E., Aznar, R., Gomez-Arzapalo, E., Pascual, C., and Giner, J.: Correlation between sperm motility and electrolyte composition of seminal fluid in normal and infertile men. Fertil. Steril., *24*:150, 1973.

26. Borkovec, A. B.: Methotrexate as an insect sterilant. Science, 37:1034, 1962.
27. Brown, F. T., and Osgood, A. T.: X-rays and sterility. Amer. J. Surg., 18:179, 1905.
28. Bydgeman, M., Fredricson, K., Svanborg, K., and Samuelson, B.: The relation between fertility and prostaglandin content of seminal fluid in man. Fertil. Steril., 21:622, 1970.
29. de la Calancha, A.: Cronica Moralizada de La Orden De San Agustin: Barcelona, Pedro Lacabelleria, 1639.
30. Chang, M. C.: Disintegration of epididymal spermatozoa by application of ice to the scrotal testis. J. Exp. Biol., 20:16, 1943.
31. Charny, C. W., and Wolgin, W.: Cryptorchism. New York, Paul B. Hoeber, Inc., 1957.
32. Cognat, M., and Guillaud, M.: The artificial spermatocele in cases with congenital aplasia of sperm duct. Andrologia, 5:37, 1973.
33. Collier, J. G., and Flower, R. J.: Effect of aspirin on human seminal prostaglandins. Lancet, 2:852, 1971.
34. Coombs, R. R. A., Rümke, P., and Edwards, R. G.: Immunoglobulin classes reactive with spermatozoa in the serum and seminal plasma of vasectomized and infertile men. In Bratanov, K.·(ed.): Second International Symposium on Immunology of Reproduction. Sofia, Bulgaria, Bulgerian Academy of Sciences Press, 1972.
35. DeLouvois, J., Harrison, R. F., Blades, M., Hurley, R., and Stanley, V. C.: Frequency of mycoplasma in fertile and infertile couples. Lancet, 1:1074, 1974.
35a. Dieckmann, W. J., Davis, M. E., Rynkeiwicz, S. M., and Pottinger, R. E.: Does the administration of diethylstilbestrol during pregnancy have therapeutic value? Amer. J. Obstet. Gynecol., 66:1062, 1953.
36. Dienes, L., and Edsall, J.: Observations on the L-organism of Kleineberger. Proc. Soc. Exp. Biol. Med., 36:740, 1937.
37. Dmowsky, W. P., Scholer, H. F. L., Mahesh, V. B., and Greenblatt, R. B.: Danazol—a synthetic steroid derivative with interesting physiologic properties. Fertil. Steril., 22:9, 1971.
38. Dokov, V., and Timmermanns, L.: Arrest of spermatogenesis by certain antibiotics. Acta Urol. Belg., 38:277, 1970.
39. Drake, T., and Mailbach, H.: Taking the heartbreak out of psoriasis. Mod. Med., 43:90, 1975.
40. Ellis, L. C., Hargrove, L. L., Johnson, J. M. et al.: Prostaglandins and the dual endocrine role of the testis. Res. Reprod., 4:2, 1972.
41. Engle, E. T.: The testis and hormones. In Cowdry, E. V. (ed.): Problems of Aging. Baltimore, The Williams & Wilkins Co., 1942.
42. Ericsson, R. J.: Chemosterilants. In Sciarra, J. J., Markland, C., and Speidel, J. J. (eds.): Control of Male Fertility. Hagerstown, Maryland, Harper and Row, 1975.
43. Fairley, K. F., Barrie, J. U., and Johnson, W.: Sterility and testicular atrophy related to cyclophosphamide therapy. Lancet, 1:568, 1972.
44. Fjallbrant, B.: Interrelation between high levels of sperm antibodies, reduced penetration of cervical mucus by spermatozoa and sterility in men. Acta Obstet. Gynecol. Scand., 47:102, 1968.
45. Fowlkes, D. M., Dooher, G. B., and O'Leary, W. M.: Evidence by scanning electron microscopy for an association between human spermatozoa and T-mycoplasmas in men of infertile marriage. Fertil. Steril., 26:1203, 1975.
46. Fowlkes, D. M., MacLeod, J., and O'Leary, W. M.: T-mycoplasmas and human infertility: correlation of infection with alterations in seminal parameters. Fertil. Steril., 26:1212, 1975.
47. Franklin, R. R., and Dukes, C. D.: Antispermatozoal antibody and unexplained infertility. Amer. J. Obstet. Gynecol., 89:6, 1964.
48. Franklin, R. R., and Dukes, C. D.: Antispermatozoal antibody and unexplained infertility, further studies. J.A.M.A., 190:682, 1964.
49. Frehn, J. L., Urry, R. L., Balph, D. F., et al.: Photo-period and crowding effects on testicular serotonin metabolism and lack of effects on melatonin synthesis in Uinta ground squirrels. J. Exp. Zool., 183:139, 1973.
50. French, D. J., Leeb, C. S., and Jecht, E. W.: Reduction in sperm output by febrile attacks of familial Mediterranean fever. A case report. Fertil. Steril., 24:490, 1973.
51. Freund, M.: Effect of frequency of emission on semen output and an estimate of daily sperm production in man. J. Reprod. Fertil., 8:149, 1964.

52. Friberg, J., and Gnarpe, H.: Mycoplasmas in semen from fertile and infertile men. Andrologia, 6:45, 1974.
53. Fukui, N.: On a hitherto unknown action of heat rays on testicles. Jap. Med. World, 3:27, 1923.
54. Gassner, F., and Hopwood, M. L.: Seminal amino acids and carbohydrate pattern of bulls with normal and abnormal testis function. Proc. Soc. Exp. Biol. Med., 81:37, 1952.
55. Giarola, A., and Agostini, G.: Amino acids in the treatment of male sterility. In Westin, B., and Wiqvist, N. (eds.): Proceedings of the Fifth World Congress on Fertility and Sterility, Stockholm, June 16–22, 1966. Amsterdam, Excerpta Medica Foundation, 1967, p. 892.
56. Giarola, A.: Protection of reproductive capacity as a factor in therapy for undescended testicle. Fertil. Steril., 18:375, 1967.
56a. Gill, W. B., Schumacher, G. F. B., and Bibbo, M.: Structural and functional abnormalities in the sex organs of male offspring of mothers treated with diethylstilbestrol (DES). J. Reprod. Med., 16:147, 1976.
57. Gnarpe, H., and Friberg, J.: Mycoplasma and human reproductive failure. 1. The occurrences of different mycoplasmas in couples with reproductive failure. Amer. J. Obstet. Gynecol., 114:727, 1972.
58. Gnarpe, H., and Griberg, J.: T-mycoplasmas on spermatozoa and infertility. Nature, 245:97, 1973.
59. Grayhack, J. T., and Scott, W. W.: The effect of general and dietary deficiencies and response of the prostate of the albino rat to testosterone proprionate. Endocrinology, 50:406, 1952.
60. Greenblatt, R. B., Dmowski, W. P., Mahesh, V. B., and Scholer, H. F. L.: Clinical studies with an anti-gonadotrophin, Danazol. Fertil. Steril., 22:10, 1971.
60a. Greenwald, P., Barlow, J. J., Nasca, P. C., and Barnett, W. S.: Vaginal cancer after maternal treatment with synthetic estrogens. N. Engl. J. Med., 285:309, 1971.
61. Halpern, B. N., Ky, T., and Robert, B.: Clinical and immunological study of an exceptional case of reagenic type sensitization to human seminal fluid. Immunology, 12:247, 1967.
62. Hanley, H. G.: The surgery of male sub-fertility. Ann. R. Coll. Surg. Engl., 17:159, 1955.
63. Hanley, H. G.: Pregnancy following artifical insemination from epididymal cyst. Studies on fertility. Proc. Soc. Stud. Fertil., 8:20, 1956.
64. Harris, R., and Harrison, R. G.: The effect of low temperature on the guinea pig testis. Studies on Fertility, 7:23, 1955.
65. Hartman, C. G.: Science and the Safe Period. Baltimore, The Williams & Wilkins Co., 1962.
66. Hecker, W. C., and Hienz, H. A.: Cryptorchism and fertility. J. Pediatr. Surg., 2:513, 1967.
67. Hekman, A., and Rümke, P. H.: The antigens of human seminal plasma with special reference to lactoferrin as a spermatozoa-coating antigen. Fertil. Steril., 20:312, 1969.
68. Heller, C. G., Moore, D. J., and Paulsen, C. A.: Suppression of spermatogenesis and chronic toxicity in man by a new series of bis (dichloracetyl) diamines. Toxicol. Appl. Pharmacol., 3:1, 1960.
69. Heller, C. G., Morse, H. C., Su, U., and Rowley, M. J.: The role of FSH, ICSH and endogenous testosterone during testicular suppression by exogenous testosterone in normal men. In Rosenberg, E., and Paulsen, C. A. (eds.): Human Testis. New York, Plenum Press, 1970, pp. 249–257.
69a. Herbst, A. L., Robboy, S. J., Scully, R. E., and Poskanzer, D. C.: Clear-cell adenocarcinoma of the vagina and cervix in girls: analyses of 170 registry cases. Amer. J. Obstet. Gynecol., 119:713, 1974.
69b. Herbst, A. L., and Scully, R. E.: Adenocarcinoma of the vagina in adolescence: a report of seven cases including six clear-cell carcinomas (so-called mesonephromas). Cancer, 25:745, 1970.
70. Horne, H. W., Jr., and Maddock, C. L.: Vitamin A therapy in oligospermia. Fertil. Steril., 3:245, 1952.
71. Horne, H. W., Kundsin, R. B., and Kosasa, T. S.: The role of mycoplasma infection in human reproductive failure. Fertil. Steril., 25:380, 1974.
72. Hotchkiss, R. S.: Review: the human testis. Fertil. Steril., 7:284, 1956.

73. Hulka, J. F., and Davis, J. E.: Vasectomy and reversible vasocclusion. Fertil. Steril., 23:683, 1972.
74. Ishigami, J.: Non-endocrine drugs in the treatment of male infertility. Amsterdam, Excerpta Medica, Int. Congr. Ser. 109, 1966.
75. Isojima, S., Li, T. S., and Ashitaka, Y.: Immunological analysis of sperm-immobilizing factor found in sera of women with unexplained infertility. Amer. J. Obstet. Gynecol., 101:677, 1968.
76. Jackson, H., Fox, B. W., and Craig, A. W.: Antifertility substances and their assessment in the male rodent. J. Reprod. Fertil., 2:447, 1961.
77. Jackson, H., Partington, M., and Fox, B. W.: Effect of busulphan (Myleran) on the spermatogenic cell population of the rat testis. Nature, 194:1184, 1962.
78. Janick, J., Zeitz, L., and Whitmore, W. F.: Seminal fluid and spermatozoan zinc levels and their relationship to human spermatozoan motility. Fertil. Steril., 22:573, 1971.
79. Johnson, M. H.: The distribution of immunoglobulin and spermatozoal auto-antigen in the genital tract of the male guinea pig. Its relationship to autoallergic orchitis. Fertil. Steril., 23:383, 1972.
80. Jubiz, W., and Frailey, J.: Seminal fluid and plasma prostaglandin responses to aspirin in normal subjects. Fertil. Steril., 24:977, 1973.
81. Kibrick, S., Belding, D. L., and Merrill, B.: Methods for the detection of antibodies against mammalian spermatozoa. II. A gelatin agglutination test. Fertil. Steril., 3:430, 1952.
82. Kirsh, I. E.: Radiation dangers in diagnostic radiology. J.A.M.A., 158:1420, 1955.
83. Kolodny, R. C., Masters, W. H., Kolodner, R. M., et al.: Depression of plasma testosterone levels after chronic intensive marihuana use. N. Engl. J. Med., 290:872, 1974.
84. Kolansky, H., and Moore, W. T.: Marihuana, can it hurt you? J.A.M.A., 232:923, 1975.
85. Krahn, H. P., Tessler, A. N., and Hotchkiss, R. S.: Studies on effect of hydrocele on scrotal temperature, pressure and testicular morphology. Fertil. Steril., 14:226, 1963.
86. Kumar, A., Bagghi, S. C., and Indrayan, A.: Impact of lepromatous leprosy on fecundity. Fertil. Steril., 24:324, 1973.
87. Kumar, A., Biggart, J. D., McEvoy, J., and McGeown, M. G.: Cyclophosphamide and reproductive function. Lancet, 1:1212, 1972.
88. Kupperman, H. S., and Epstein, J. A.: Endocrine therapy of sterility. Amer. Prac., 9:547, 1958.
89. Lancranjan, I., Popescu, H. I., Gavanescu, O., Klepsch, I., and Servanescu, M.: Reproductive ability of workmen occupationally exposed to lead. Arch. Environ. Health, 30:396, 1975.
90. Lattimer, J. K., Colmore, H. P., Sanger, G., Robertson, D. H., and McLellan, F. C.: Transmission of genital tuberculosis from husband to wife via semen. Amer. Rev. Tuberc., 69:618, 1954.
91. Lattimer, J. K., Uson, A. C., and Melicow, M. M.: Tuberculous infections and inflammations. In Campbell, M. E., and Harrison, J. H. (eds.): Urology. 3rd ed. Philadelphia, W. B. Saunders Co., 1963, p. 417–418.
92. Leathem, J. H.: Nutritional effects in endocrine secretions. In Young, W. C. (ed.): Sex and Internal Secretions. Baltimore, The Williams & Wilkins Co., 1962, p. 666–704.
93. Leblond, C. P., Steinberger, E., and RoosenRunge, E. C.: Spermatogenesis. In Hartman, C. G. (ed.): Mechanisms Concerned with Conception. New York, Macmillan Co., 1963.
94. Levine, B. B., Siraganian, R. P., and Schenkein, I.: Allergy to human seminal plasma. N. Engl. J. Med., 288:894, 1973.
95. Lindahl, P. E., and Kihlström, J. E.: An antiagglutinic factor in mammalian sperm plasma. Fertil. Steril., 5:241, 1954.
96. Lindholmer, C.: Toxicity of zinc ions to human spermatozoa and the influence of albumin. Andrologia, 6:7, 1974.
97. Lindholmer, C., and Eliasson, R.: The effects of albumin, magnesium and zinc on human sperm survival in different fractions of the split ejaculate. Fertil. Steril., 25:424, 1974.
98. Lipshultz, L. I.: Cryptorchidism in the subfertile male. Fertil. Steril., 27:609, 1976.
99. Lipshultz, L. I., Caminos-Torres, R., Greenspan, C. S., and Snyder, P. J.: Testicular

function after orchiopexy for unilaterally undescended testis. N. Engl. J. Med., *295*:15, 1976.

100. Lui, C-C., and Kinson, G. A.: Testicular gametogenic and endocrine responses to melatonin and serotonin peripherally administered to mature rats. Contraception, *7*:153, 1973.
101. Lutwak-Mann, C.: Dependence of gonadal function upon vitamins and other nutritional factors. Vitam. Horm., *16*:35, 1958.
102. McCormack, W. M., Almeida, P. C., Bailey, P. B., Grady, E. M., and Lee, Y. H.: Sexual activity and vaginal colinization with genital mycoplasmas. J.A.M.A., *221*:1375, 1972.
103. McCormack, W. M., Braun, P., Lee, Y. H., Klein, J. O., and Kass, E. H.: The genital mycoplasmas. N. Engl. J. Med., *288*:78, 1973.
104. McCoy, W. G.: Fecundity of the Hawaiian lepers. Publ. Health Bull., *61*:23, 1913.
105. MacDonald, J., and Harrison, R. G.: Effect of low temperature on rat spermatogenesis. Fertil. Steril., *5*:205, 1954.
106. MacLeod, J.: Effect of chicken pox and pneumonia on semen quality. Fertil. Steril., *2*:523, 1951.
107. MacLeod, J.: Studies in human spermatogenesis: the effect of certain anti-spermatogenic compounds. Anat. Rec., *139*:250, 1961.
108. MacLeod, J.: Testicular response during and following severe allergic reaction. Fertil. Steril., *13*:531, 1962.
109. MacLeod, J.: Human seminal cytology as a sensitive indicator of the germinal epithelium. Int. J. Fertil., *9*:281, 1964.
110. MacLeod, J., and Hotchkiss, R. S.: The effect of hyperexia upon spermatozoa counts in men. Endocrinology, *28*:780, 1941.
111. MacLeod, J., Hotchkiss, R. S., and Sitterson, B. W.: Recovery of male fertility after sterilization by nuclear radiation. J.A.M.A., *187*:637, 1964.
112. Mancini, R. E.: Immunological aspects of male infertility. *In* Rosenberg, E., and Paulsen, C. A. (eds.): The Human Testis. New York, Plenum Press, 1970.
113. Mancini, R. E., Andrada, J. A., Seraceni, D., Bachman, A. E., Lavieri, J. C., and Nemirovsky, M.: Immunological and testicular response in man sensitized with human testicular homogenate. J. Clin. Endocrinol., *25*:859, 1965.
114. Mann, R.: The Biochemistry of Semen and of the Male Reproductive Tract. New York, John Wiley and Sons, 1964.
115. Mardh, P. A., and Westrom, L.: T-myocplasmas in the genitoruinary tract of the female. Acta Path. Microbiol. Scand., *78*:367, 1970.
116. Martin-Delson, P. A., Shaver, E., and Gammal, E. B.: Chromosome abnormalities in rabbit blastocysts resulting from spermatozoa aged in the male tract. Fertil. Steril., *24*:212, 1973.
117. Mason, K. E.: Relation of vitamins to sex glands. *In* Allen, E., Denforth, C. H., and Dorsey, E. A. (eds.): Sex and Internal Secretions. Baltimore, The Williams & Wilkins Co., 1939, p. 1149.
118. Merlin, H. E.: Azoospermia caused by colchicine—a case report. Fertil. Steril., *23*:180, 1972.
119. Metchnikoff, E.: Études sur la resorption des cellules. Ann. Int. Pasteur, *13*:737, 1899.
120. Mineberg, D., and Bingol, N.: Chromosomal abnormalities in undescended testes. Urology, *1*:98, 1973.
121. Monge, C., and Mori-Charez, P.: Fisiologia de la reproduccion en la altura. Le espermatogenesis en la altura. An. Fac. Med. Lima, *25*:34, 1942.
122. Moore, C. R., and Samuels, L. T.: The action of testis hormone in correcting changes induced in the rat prostate and seminal vesicles by vitamin B deficiency or partial inanition. Amer. J. Physiol., *96*:278, 1931.
123. Morales, P. A., and Harden, J.: Scrotal and testicular temperature studies in paraplegics. J. Urol., *79*:972, 1958.
124. Mroueh, A.: Effect of arginine in oligospermia. Fertil. Steril., *21*:217, 1970.
125. Mumford, D. M., Barsales, P. B., Ball, K. D., and Gorden, H. L.: Microlymphocyte transformation studies with seminal antigen. I. Technique and patterns of responsiveness to autologous and allogenic semen from normal and infertile male subjects. J. Urol., *105*:858, 1971.
126. Nahas, C. G.: When friends or patients ask about marihuana. J.A.M.A., *233*:79, 1975.

127. Nelson, W. O., and Steinberger, E.: The effect of furadoxyl upon the testis of the rat. Anat. Rec., *112*:367, 1952.
128. Nelson, W. O., and Bunge, R. G.: The effect of therapeutic dosages of nitrofurantoin (Furadantin) upon spermatogenesis in man. J. Urol., 77:275, 1965.
129. Newman, H. F., and Wilhelm, S. F.: Testicular temperature in man. J. Urol., *63*:349, 1950.
130. Nilsson, S., Obrant, K. O., and Persson, P. S.: Changes in the testis parenchyma caused by acute non-specific epididymitis. Fertil. Steril., *19*:748, 1968.
131. Oakberg, E. F.: Initial depletion and subsequent recovery of spermatogonia of the mouse after 20 r of gamma rays and 100, 300, and 600 r of x-rays. Radiat. Res., *11*:700, 1959.
132. Pancheco-Romero, J. C., Gleich, G. J., Loegering, D. A., and Johnson, C. E.: Spermagglutinating activity and female infertility. J.A.M.A., *224*:849, 1973.
133. Parker, R. G., and Holyoke, B.: Tumors of the testis. Amer. J. Roentgenol., *83*:43, 1960.
134. Patton, W. C., and Taymor, M. L.: An investigation of the relationship between cervical mycoplasma infection, the postcoital test, and infertility. Fertil. Steril., *26*:211, 1975.
135. Perez, I. R., and Prendes, M. A. G.: Orgutis epididimitis of otros factores que dimniuyen fa fecundidad en los sujetros leprosons. Rev. Sif. Leprol. Derm., *1*:20, 1944.
136. Phadke, A. M., and Padukone, K.: Presence and significance of auto-antibodies against spermatozoa in the blood of men with obstructed vas deferens. J. Reprod. Fertil., 7:163, 1964.
137. Phadke, A. M., Samant, N. R., and Dewal, S. D.: Smallpox as an etiologic factor in male infertility. Fertil. Steril., *24*:802, 1973.
138. Poffenbarger, P. L., Brinkley, B. R., and Goldfinger, S. E.: Colchicine for familial Mediterranean fever: possible adverse effects. N. Engl. J. Med., *290*:56, 1974.
139. Potts, G. O., Beyler, A. L., and Schane, H. P.: Pituitary gonadotropin inhibitory activity of Danazol. Fertil. Steril., *25*:367, 1974.
140. Prior, J., and Ferguson, J.: Cytoxic effects of a nitrofuran on the rat testis. Cancer, *3*:62, 1950.
141. Quesada, E. M., Dukes, C. D., Deem, G. H., and Franklin, R. R.: Genital infections and sperm agglutinating antibodies in infertile men. J. Urol., 99:106, 1968.
142. Rao, S. S., and Sadri, K. K.: Proceedings of the Sixth International Conference on Planned Parenthood. New Delhi, 1959, p. 243.
143. Regand, C., and Dubreuil, G.: Action des rayons de roentgen sur la testicule de lapin. Conservation de la puissance virile et stérilisation. Compt. Rend. Soc. Biol., *63*:647, 1907.
144. Richter, P., Calamera, J. C., Morgenfeld, M. C., Kierszenbaum, A. L., Lavieri, J. C., and Mancini, R. E.: Effect of chlorambucil on spermatogenesis in the human with malignant lymphoma. Cancer, *25*:1026, 1970.
145. Robinson, D., and Rock, J.: Intrascrotal hyperthermia induced by scrotal insulation; effect on spermatogenesis. Obstet. Gynecol., *29*:217, 1967.
146. Robinson, D., and Rock, J.: Control of human spermatogenesis by induced changes of intrascrotal temperature. J.A.M.A., *204*:290, 1968.
147. Rock, J., and Robinson, D.: Effect of induced intrascrotal hyperthermia on testicular function in man. Amer. J. Obstet. Gynecol., *93*:793, 1965.
148. Rock, J., Titze, C., McLaughlin, H. B.: Effect of adoption on infertility. Fertil. Steril., *16*:305, 1965.
149. Roenigk, H., Mailbach, H., and Weinstein, G.: Methotrexate therapy for psoriasis: guideline revisions. Arch. Dermatol., *108*:35, 1973.
150. Roosen-Runge, E. C.: Quantitative studies on spermatogenesis in the albino rat. II. The duration of spermatogenesis and some effects of colchicine. Amer. J. Anat., *88*:163, 1951.
151. Rosada, A., Hicks, J. J., Martinez-Zedillo, G., *et al.:* Inhibitions of human sperm motility by calcium and zinc ions. Conception, *2*:259, 1970.
152. Ross, V., Moore, D. H., and Miller, E. G.: Proteins of human seminal plasma. J. Biol. Chem., *144*:667, 1942.
153. Rubin, L.: Sexual Life After Sixty. New York, Basic Books, Inc., 1965.
154. Rümke, P.: The presence of sperm antibodies in the serum of two patients with oligospermia. Vox. Sang., *4*:135, 1954.

155. Rümke, P.: Sperm agglutinating autoantibodies in relation to male infertility. Proc. R. Soc. Med., 61:275, 1968.
156. Rümke, P.: Autoantibodies against spermatozoa in infertile men. J. Reprod. Fertil. (Suppl.), 21:169, 1974.
157. Rümke, P., and Hellinga, G.: Autoantibodies against spermatozoa in sterile men. Amer. J. Clin. Pathol., 32:357, 1959.
158. Rümke, P., Van Amstel, N., Messer, E. N., et al.: Prognosis of fertility of men with sperm agglutinins in the serum. Fertil. Steril., 25:393, 1974.
159. Salvatierra, O., Jr., Fortzmann, J. L., and Belzer, F. O.: Sexual function in males before and after renal transplantation. Urology, 5:64, 1975.
160. Sand, K.: Die Physiologie des Hodens. Leipzig, 1933.
161. Sandler, B.: Conception after adoption: a comparision of conception rates. Fertil. Steril., 16:313, 1965.
162. Schacter, A., Goldman, J. A., and Zuckerman, Z.: Treatment of oligospermia with the amino acid arginine. J. Urol., 110:311, 1973.
163. Schoysman, R. J.: La creation d'un spermatocele artificiel dans les argenesies du canal deferent. Bull. Soc. R. Belge. Gynecol. Obstet., 38:307, 1968.
164. Schoysman, R. J.: Surgical treatment of obstructive azoospermia. An unpublished report presented at the annual meeting of the Pacific Coast Fertility Society in Palm Springs, California, October 27, 1973.
165. Schoysman, R. J., and Drouart, J. M.: Progres recents dans la chirurgie de la sterilite masculine et feminine. Acta Chir. Belg., 71:261, 1972.
166. Scorer, C. G.: The descent of the testis. Arch. Dis. Child., 39:605, 1964.
167. Scorer, C. G., and Farrington, G. H.: Congenital Deformities of the Testis and Epididymis. London, Butterworth and Co., 1971, Chapters 5 and 6.
168. Scott, L. S.: Delayed treatment of cryptorchism and subsequent infertility. Fertil. Steril., 18:782, 1967.
169. Segal, S., Sadovsky, E., Palti, Z., Pfeifer, Y., and Polishuk, W. Z.: Serotonin and 5-hydroxyindoleacetic acid (5-HIAA) in fertile and subfertile men. Fertil. Steril., 26:314, 1975.
170. Serreira, N. R., and Buoniconti, A.: Trisomy after colchicine therapy. Lancet, 2:1304, 1968.
171. Seymour, F. I., Duffy, C., and Koerner, A.: A case of authenticated fertility in a man of 94. J.A.M.A., 105:1423, 1935.
172. Sherins, R. J., and DeVita, V. T., Jr.: Effect of drug treatment for lymphoma on male reproductive capacity. Studies in men in remission after therapy. Ann. Intern. Med., 79:216, 1973.
173. Shulman, S.: Immunity and infertility. A review. Contraception, 4:135, 1971.
174. Shulman, S.: Sperm antibodies as a cause of infertility. CRC Crit. Rev. Clin. Lab. Sci., 2:393, 1971.
175. Shulman, S., Zappi, E., Ahmed, U., et al.: Immunologic consequence of vasectomy. Contraception, 5:269, 1972.
176. Skoglund, R. D., and Paulsen, C. A.: Danazol–testosterone combination: a potentially effective means for reversible male contraception. A preliminary report. Contraception, 7:357, 1973.
177. Stadtler, F., and Horn, H. J.: Changes in human testes during anti-androgen treatment: histologic morphologic, and enzyme-histochemical studies of testicular biopsies. Dtsch. Med. Wochenschr., 98:1013, 1973.
177a. Stafl, A., Mattingly, R. F., Foley, D. V., and Fetherstron, W. C.: Clinical diagnosis of vaginal adenosis. Obstet. Gynecol., 43:118, 1974.
178. Steinberger, E.: A radiometric effect of triethylenemelamine on reproduction in the male rat. Endocrinol., 65:40, 1959.
179. Stemmerman, G. N., Weiss, L., Auerbach, O., and Friedman, M.: A study of the germinal epithelium in male paraplegics. Amer. J. Clin. Pathol., 20:24, 1950.
180. Stewart, B. H.: Personal communication, 1976.
181. Stewart-Bentley, M., Vergi, A., Chang, S., Hiatt, R., and Horton, R.: Effects of Dilantin on FSH and spermatogenesis. Clin. Res., 24:101, 1976.
182. Stieve, H.: Kastration durch Hitze mit nachfolgender Wucherung des Keimepithels. Z. Mikrosk. Anat. Forsch., 1:191, 1924.
183. Talbot, H. W.: A report on sexual function in paraplegics. J. Urol., 61:265, 1949.

184. Tanimura, J.: Studies on arginine in human semen. Part III. The influence of several drugs on male infertility. Bull. Osaka Med. Sch., *13*:90, 1967.
185. Taylor-Robinson, D., and Manchee, R. J.: Mycoplasma Diseases of Man. Jena, Gustav Fischer Verlag, 1969, p. 113.
186. Taylor-Robinson, D., Thomas, M., and Dawson, P. L. J.: The isolation of T-mycoplasmas from the urogenital tract of bulls. J. Med. Microbiol., *2*:527, 1969.
187. Teague, N. S., Boyarsky, S., and Glenn, J. F.: Interference of human spermatozoa motility by *Escherichia coli*. Fertil. Steril., *22*:281, 1971.
188. Terry, L. B.: Smoking and Health. Report of the Advisory Committee to the Surgeon General of the Public Health Service. Public Health Service Publ. No. 1103. Washington, D.C., U.S. Govt. Print. Off., 1964.
189. Thurm, J.: Sexual potency of patients on chronic hemodialysis. Urology, *5*:60, 1975.
190. Timmermans, L.: Influence of antibiotics on spermatogenesis. J. Urol., *112*:348, 1974.
191. Tourville, D. R., Orga, S. S., Lippes, J., and Tomasi, T. B., Jr.: The human female reproductive tract: immunohistochemical localization of AGM secretory "piece" and lactoferrin. Amer. J. Obstet. Gynecol., *108*:1102, 1970.
192. Tyler, A., and Bishop, D.: Immunological phenomena. *In* Hartman, C. G. (ed.): Mechanisms Concerned with Conception. New York, Macmillan Co., 1963, pp. 397–482.
193. Urry, R. L., and Dougherty, K. A.: Inhibition of rat spermatogenesis and seminiferous tubule growth after short-term and long-term administration of monoamine oxidase inhibitor. Fertil. Steril., *26*:232, 1975.
194. Vickers, M. A., Jr.: Creation and use of a scrotal sperm bank in aplasia of the vas deferens. J. Urol., *114*:242, 1975.
195. Von Lanz, T.: Beobachtungen und Versuche am Nebenhoden der Hausmaus. Z. Anat. Entwicklungsgesch., *74*:761, 1924.
196. Walker, K.: The critical age in men. Sexology, *30*:705, 1964.
197. Walsh, P. C., and Swerdloff, R. S.: Biphasic effect of testosterone on spermatogenesis in the rat. Invest. Urol., *11*:190, 1973.
198. Weir, W. C., and Weir, D. R.: Adoption and subsequent conception. Fertil. Steril., *17*:283, 1966.
199. White, I. G.: The toxicity of heavy metals to mammalian spermatozoa. Aust. J. Exp. Biol. Med. Sci., *33*:359, 1955.
200. Wilson, L.: Sperm agglutinins in human semen and blood. Proc. Soc. Exp. Biol. Med., *85*:642, 1954.
201. Wilson, L.: Sperm agglutination due to autoantibodies. A new cause for sterility. Fertil. Steril., *7*:262, 1956.
202. Young, W. C.: The influence of high temperature on the guinea pig testis: histological changes and effects on reproduction. J. Exp. Zool., *49*:459, 1927.
203. Zappi, E., Ahmen, U., Davis, J., *et al.:* Immunologic consequences of vasectomy. Fed. Proc., *29*:729, 1970.

Part *II*

DIAGNOSTIC MEASURES

Chapter 5

SEMEN ANALYSIS

RICHARD D. AMELAR, M.D.
LAWRENCE DUBIN, M.D.

The semen analysis must be considered the most important single item in the evaluation of male fertility. Since some variation occurs normally, at least two specimens should be examined before any judgment of impaired fertility is made.

HISTORY

In the early seventeenth century Antoni Van Leeuwenhoek, a dry goods clerk in Amsterdam, took up the hobby of grinding microscope lenses and was able to achieve a magnification of 370 diameters. His young

105

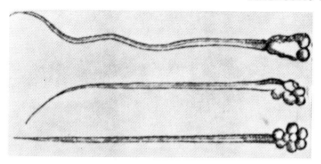

Figure 5–1. Sketches of spermatozoa as seen by Leeuwenhoek. (From Philosophical Transactions of the Royal Society of London, 1677.)

associate, Hamm, using one of these lenses, saw spermatozoa for the first time. To quote from Leeuwenhoek's letter to the Royal Society of London in November 1677, Hamm saw "living animalcules in human semen, judging these to possess tails... sometimes more than a thousand were moving in an amount of material the size of a grain of sand"[15] (Fig. 5–1). Other microscopists described miniature parts of the body within the sperm head, including the "homunculus" (little man), which was pictured in woodcuts published in the Philosophical Transactions of the Royal Society of London in 1678 (Fig. 5–2). Leeuwenhoek believed that sperm developed directly into an animal or human being, and to his dying day had no use for an egg. Leeuwenhoek was also the first to describe spermine phosphate crystals in semen which "had stood for a little while" (Fig. 5–3).

The origin of semen analysis can be traced back to the invention of the compound microscope. Spallanzani performed the first quantitative studies

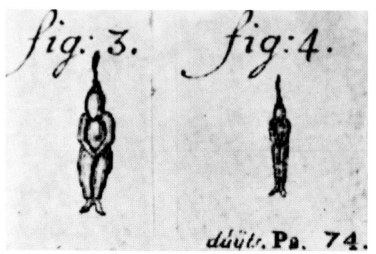

Figure 5–2. Spermatozoa were conceived as "little men" or homunculi by some microscopists toward the end of the seventeenth century. (From Philosophical Transactions of the Royal Society of London, 1678.)

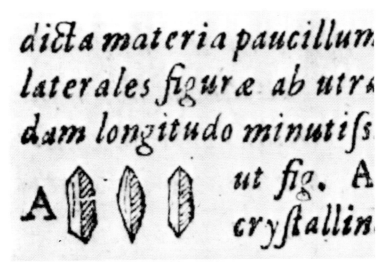

Figure 5-3. Spermine phosphate crystals in human semen as seen by Leeuwenhoek in 1677. (From Philosophical Transactions of the Royal Society of London, 1678.)

on the seminal fluid of amphibia in 1780.[53] The assessment of the sperm density in relation to human fertility was first employed by gynecologists through the examination of postcoital vaginal and cervical fluids. The first report of such an examination must be credited to Donne in 1844, who found spermatozoa in the vaginal mucus of a patient in whom he was studying the mucosa of the vagina and uterus.[9]

In 1866, the first true postcoital examination for clinical reasons was performed by Sims.[45] The first count of spermatozoa, basically as we know it today, was performed by Macomber and Sanders in 1929.[38] They concluded that pregnancies could occur with sperm counts of less than 60 million per milliliter, but higher counts were believed to increase the chances of a pregnancy.

COLLECTION OF THE SPECIMEN

The specimen of semen should be collected directly into a supplied clean, dry glass or plastic wide-mouthed container by masturbation or coitus interruptus after a period of abstinence corresponding to the couple's usual coital frequency. Such timing has greater clinical significance than an artificial standard of, for instance, 3 to 5 days because it portrays more accurately the character of the ejaculate being presented to the female generative tract. On receipt of the semen specimen in the laboratory, notation is made of the time of collection and the period of abstinence prior to collection.

The patient must be cautioned to be certain that the entire semen specimen is placed within the bottle and that no portion of it is lost. Since the distribution of sperm cells is not uniform throughout the entire ejaculate, loss of the first or last portion may give entirely erroneous results.

It is usually best for the patient to collect the specimen in his own home and deliver it to the examiner within 2 hours of its collection. If the patient lives at a considerable distance from the place of examination, the specimen can be collected in a private area of the doctor's office, although this procedure may sometimes be psychologically embarrassing to the patient.

A condom should not be used for the collection of a semen specimen because the sperm-immobilizing properties of the materials used in its manufacture will interfere with any evaluation of sperm motility.

For Catholic patients whose beliefs proscribe the collection of a semen specimen by masturbation or coitus interruptus, we supply a plastic condom-type seminal pouch.* This pouch is applied to the penis in condom fashion and held in place with a rubber band. The patient can perforate it in accordance with the dictates of his conscience. To minimize the loss of semen, the hole should be made with a pin and not be placed at the bottom of the sheath. Normal sperm motility is maintained for long periods in this plastic device. The whole sheath is carefully removed by the patient after ejaculation and placed in the jar for delivery to the examiner to minimize any loss of the seminal fluid before it arrives at the laboratory.

The method of sperm collection and examination for Catholic patients advocated by T. H. Johnson[23] is mentioned only to be condemned. Johnson suggests that a drop of residual semen be collected by the patient from the urethra immediately after intercourse, placed on a slide within a circle of petroleum jelly, and delivered as a "slide sandwich" to the laboratory for examination. Since such a specimen represents, in fact, the last drops of the second part of a split ejaculate, and since most of the better quality sperm are usually in the first portion of the ejaculate, the results obtained by such an examination would be unreliable and misleading.

The strictly orthodox Jewish patient may present even more of a problem than the devout Catholic in the collection of a semen specimen.[14] (For further consideration of dealing with the obstacles posed by orthodox Jewish law in treating patients with infertility problems, see Chapter 10.) Occasionally there are patients who will not collect a semen specimen under any circumstances, and in such instances one must resort to the postcoital test for semen collection.

This raises the question of why a semen examination is necessary if a good postcoital test is available. The reason is that abnormal sperm structure may play a significant role in male infertility, and sperm motility and seminal cytology cannot be evaluated properly by a postcoital test. In addition, the volume of the seminal ejaculum may suggest to the urologist

---

*Obtainable from Milex Products, Chicago, Illinois, 60631, at a cost of about 90 cents.

various therapeutic possibilities; measurement of semen volume cannot be made in the postcoital test. Furthermore, a poor result in the postcoital test does not necessarily indicate that the man is infertile because various female or immunologic factors may be involved. The postcoital test should be used as a substitute for the semen analysis only when it is impossible to persuade the patient to submit a proper specimen for examination.

CHARACTERISTICS OF SEMEN

COAGULATION AND LIQUEFACTION

The semen is ejaculated in a liquid form and becomes a gel or coagulum immediately after ejaculation, only to liquefy again within 5 to 20 minutes. The seminal fluid then remains in a viscous state, which allows the spermatozoa to achieve their full motility. The process of coagulation is enzymatic, and the substrate for the gel formation consists of a proteinlike material secreted by the seminal vesicles. The subsequent liquefaction of human semen is also an enzymatic process, catalyzed by the proteolytic enzyme present in the prostatic secretions. A liquefaction factor (LF) has been recently isolated from normal semen.[48] This factor appears to be a proteolytic enzyme with a molecular weight of 33,000. It has been demonstrated to cause the liquefaction of abnormal semen specimens that have failed to liquefy after several hours. The LF enzyme does not appear to have a true fibrinolysin activity.[49] Although this enzyme affects liquefaction, it has absolutely no effect on residual viscosity. It appears that the LF enzyme would be of clinical help in cases that demonstrate absent or poor liquefaction, although this occurs in only a fraction of 1 per cent of the specimens we have observed.

VISCOSITY

The cause of abnormally high residual viscosity of semen after it has coagulated and then liquefied remains a mystery. Viscosity is, however, a different phenomenon from coagulation,[2] and the two terms should not be confused. There is no demonstrable relationship between the proteolytic enzyme and the subsequent residual viscosity of the specimen after liquefaction.

The viscosity of the semen specimen can be adequately assessed by slowly pouring the specimen from the collection bottle into a 10 to 15 ml. graduated glass cylinder in which the volume will be measured. The seminal viscosity is usually graded on a scale of 0 (normal) to 4+. A normal specimen with a grade of 0 is capable of being poured in single, small droplets, while the 4+ specimen is a thick semisolid mass which cannot be

fractionated in pouring. Grades of 1+, 2+, and 3+ between these two extremes are judged according to the semen's capability of being poured and
fractionated into droplets. Attempts to perform sperm counts on highly viscous specimens are thwarted by the unequal concentrations of sperm cells
in different portions of the glob; we have seen sperm counts ranging from
10 million per ml. to 120 million per ml. from different portions of the same
highly viscous specimen, so that counts are likely to be inaccurate. In general, high seminal viscosity does not in itself produce fertility problems
unless it is accompanied by poor sperm motility, which is evident at microscopic examination if the sperm seem to be trapped in a mire and move
sluggishly or even vibrate in place without forward progression.

Methods of dealing with infertility problems related to delayed seminal
liquefaction and increased seminal viscosity are discussed in Chapter 10.

APPEARANCE AND ODOR

The appearance of freshly ejaculated semen is that of a grayish-white,
opalescent, gelatinous mixture. After the gel has liquefied, the semen
becomes a translucent fluid that varies from whitish to opalescent in tone,
depending on cellular content. It has a mildly acrid and distinctive odor.
An interesting psychological test has been developed along the lines of the
Rorschach test employing odors instead of visual symbols. One of the
odors used in this test is that of semen, and the patient's reactions to this
odor are noted.

VOLUME

After a period of 3 days' abstinence from sexual relations, the volume
of seminal fluid averages between 2.0 and 5.0 ml. Volumes of less than 1
ml. or more than 5 ml. are often accompanied by low sperm counts per ml.
It has been suggested that more homologous inseminations (AIH) be performed if the semen volume is 1.5 ml. or less[28] and otherwise good semen
quality and a poor postcoital test result are present. The low volume in itself may be a factor in infertility because it may not allow adequate access
of the sperm to the cervical mucus.

There is no correlation between high volumes of ejaculate and the size
or consistency of the prostate gland as judged by rectal digital examination.
It is usually not possible to obtain more than 1 ml. of secretions by prostatic massage from a patient who regularly ejaculates more than 10 ml. of
seminal fluid!

Since the split ejaculate technique may have therapeutic value in
dealing with a patient with high semen volume (see Chapter 10), the technique of collecting the split ejaculate specimen will be described here. The

patient is provided with two wide-mouthed containers which are numbered and fastened together to facilitate the collection. He is told to get the first few spurts into bottle number 1 and the remainder into bottle number 2. Ideally, the first third of the specimen should be in the first bottle and the latter two thirds in the second. The patient is advised to be careful in this process and not to readjust the volumes once the specimens have been obtained.

MICROSCOPIC EXAMINATION

The experienced observer can gain a great deal of information by simply placing a drop of semen on a glass slide and examining it under the high power of the microscope. A very good approximation of the sperm density and the type of motility and structure can be obtained. If the patient has an infection, it is usually demonstrated by the presence of a large number of pus cells. On occasion, live trichomonads or yeast cells may be found in the semen. Primitive cells of the germinal line may be confused with leukocytes by the novice observer, but these cells can be differentiated by staining with hematoxylin. This problem will be discussed in more detail later when morphology is considered.

If a specimen has been standing for some time before it is examined, large numbers of needle-shaped, colorless, spermine phosphate crystals will be noted. Chemically these are identical with Charcot-Leyden crystals (Fig. 5–4).

A forensic test used in medicolegal laboratories to identify human semen stains is based on the identification of derivatives of spermine on the material examined (such as a small piece of stained fabric). The spermine in semen comes from the prostatic secretion, and the crystals formed a few hours after ejaculation are the result of interreaction between spermine and phosphoric acid, which accumulates gradually by the action of the seminal phosphatases on organic phosphorus compounds such as phosphorylcholine.[39]

Occasionally, agglutination of the spermatozoa in the ejaculate will be noted; it may vary from occasional to severe. Three types of agglutination may occur—head to head, tail to tail, and head to tail. In most cases the agglutinated sperm appear to be motile, but the sperm cells deep inside the clumps have sluggish motility or none, and the agglutinated clumps become entangled with other clumps and with other cells and amorphous debris (Figs. 5–5 and 5–6).

A specimen without sperm cells (azoospermia) or with rare sperm cells will be immediately obvious on direct examination of a wet drop of semen. In cases when no mature sperm cells can be found, ductal obstruction can be ruled out by the careful and experienced observer, who can identify immature, round sperm precursor cells or other extraneous cells exfoliated

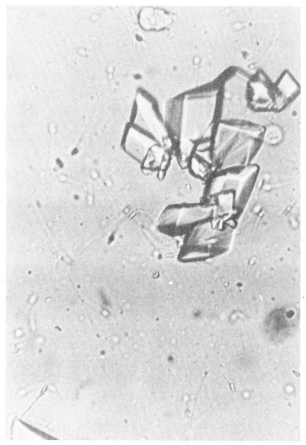

Figure 5–4. Spermine phosphate crystals. Unstained spermatozoa can be seen in the background. 150 ×

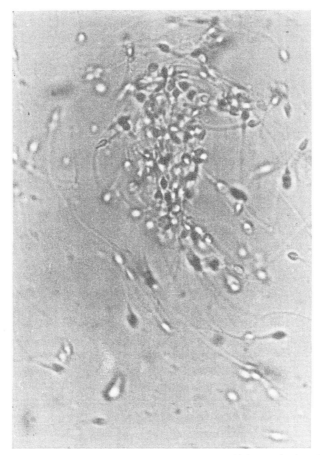

Figure 5–5. Small patch of agglutinated spermatozoa which may be found normally in specimens with a high sperm density. This amount of agglutination is not usually clinically significant.

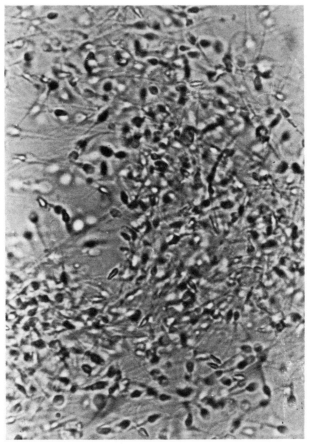

Figure 5–6. Massive agglutinated areas of spermatozoa. Head to head, tail to tail and mixed agglutination may be seen. This amount of agglutination is usually clinically significant.

from the testes.[17] Before deciding that spermatozoa or immature cells are absent from an ejaculate, the specimen should be centrifuged at 3000 rpm for 5 minutes and the sediment then reexamined, scanning a minimum of 200 high-power fields.

All azoospermic specimens should be tested for seminal fructose. Fructose is a product of the seminal vesicles and is present in all semen, with notable exceptions. It has been demonstrated that the semen of azoospermic men with congenital bilateral absence of the vas deferens and the seminal vesicles does not contain fructose and does not coagulate on ejaculation.[2] Absence of fructose is also noted in patients in whom both ejaculatory ducts are blocked.[3] In addition, fructose is absent in an unusual form of retrograde ejaculation in which a scant outward ejaculate also appears.[24] A simple qualitative test for the presence of seminal fructose will be discussed later in this chapter.

THE SPERM CELL COUNT

The sperm count is very similar to the ordinary laboratory method of performing blood cell counts. Immobilization of the sperm cells is accomplished by using a diluting fluid composed of a solution of 4 per cent sodium bicarbonate and 1 per cent phenol. (This may be prepared by mixing 16 gm. of sodium bicarbonate and 4 gm. of phenol in 400 ml. of distilled water.) A white blood cell pipette is used in combination with the red blood cell field of the standard Neubauer counting chamber; a clicker-counting device will be helpful but is not essential.

The semen specimen is thoroughly mixed, and part of it is drawn up into the white blood cell pipette. If numerous sperm cells (more than 50 per high power field) were observed when the drop of the ejaculate was examined directly, then a 1:20 dilution is made, the semen being drawn up to the 0.5 mark halfway up the stem of the pipette. The pipette is then filled to the mark at the top of its bubble-chamber with the bicarbonate-phenol solution and thoroughly shaken. On the other hand, if only a small number of sperm were observed when the semen was examined directly, a 1:10 dilution is made by drawing the semen all the way up to the 1.0 mark at the top of the stem, just below the bubble-chamber. The pipette chamber is then filled with the diluent fluid as before.

After the mixture has been thoroughly shaken, a few drops of the fluid from the stem of the pipette are discarded, and both sides of the Neubauer counting chamber (coverslip in place) are carefully filled with the pipette mixture. For greater accuracy, the count is performed twice, once on each side of the chamber, and the average is taken for computation.

The immobilized sperm cells within the red blood cell field of the counting chamber are examined, and a count is made of all sperm cells lying within five blocks of 16 small squares each (a total of 80 squares), or one fifth of the entire red blood cell field. For consistency, all cells overlying the lines at the left side and top of the squares are included in the count, and those overlying the lines at the right side and bottom are eliminated. The clicker-counter is a helpful gadget in securing the total.

The sperm cell count in millions per milliliter is then computed as follows:

1. For the 1:20 dilution, six zeros are added to the figure obtained for the total count within the five blocks.
2. For the 1:10 dilution, the total number of cells within the five-block area is divided by 2, and six zeros are added.
3. If there are very few cells in the counting chamber with the 1:10 dilution, then all the sperm cells in the entire red blood cell field are counted rather than just those in the five-block area. The number of sperm cells found in all 25 blocks is totalled, and five zeros are added to the figure obtained.

The accuracy of the count diminishes in the severely oligospermic range below 5 million per milliliter. If greater accuracy is desired in this range, 0.1 ml. of semen may be mixed with 0.1 ml. of diluting fluid and placed directly onto a counting chamber. The number of sperm counted in 25 blocks is multiplied by 2, and four zeros are added to the figure obtained.

In a study of factors affecting hemacytometer counts of sperm concentration in human semen, Freund and Carol[13] demonstrated that there is a large amount of variation among various technicians using this technique. Mean differences of about 20 per cent may be expected between duplicate determinations by the same technician; this variability must be considered as part of the inherent error in this technique and has nothing to do with the competence of the technician. For this reason, it is best to examine more than a single specimen to estimate the level of a patient's sperm production.

A bulk dilution method using large amounts of diluting fluid has also been described,[13] but it is cumbersome and impractical.

If the semen specimen is exceedingly viscous, making it difficult to draw up into the pipette, the entire specimen may be diluted in a 1:1 ratio with Alevaire to eliminate the viscosity; the resultant count is then multiplied by 2.[1]

The minimal normal value for the sperm count is not a definite figure but for our purposes can be placed around 40 million per milliliter or a total of 125 million per ejaculate, provided that the sperm motility and morphology are normal.[4] MacLeod, who has great experience, considers that true oligospermia is represented by counts of under 20 million per milliliter.[29] As long as any normal motile sperm are present, no minimum figure can be designated as the level below which pregnancy cannot be achieved. However, as the sperm count decreases, there is a corresponding decrease in the likelihood of conception, and when the sperm count is less than 10 million per milliliter it is unlikely, but not impossible, that pregnancy will occur.[41]

SPERM MOTILITY

More important than the sperm count itself is the activity or motility of the sperm cells. A drop of semen is placed on a slide and covered with a cover glass. The drop of semen should be just large enough to coat the underside of the coverslip. If it is too large, the cover glass tends to float on top of the semen, making several layers of sperm visible through the microscope and introducing the possibility of error in estimating the percentage of motile sperm. This percentage should be estimated only after many high-power fields are scanned, since there is great variation in the number of motile cells from one high-power field to another. In our laboratory a minimum of 25 high-power fields are examined before determination of the percentage of motile cells in any semen specimen is attempted.

The type of motility exhibited by the cells is classified by estimating the speed and path of their forward progression on a scale of 0 to 4. The forward motion is graded as follows[4]:

0:      No motion.
1:      Sperm moving but no forward motion visible.
1+:   Sperm moving with only slight forward motion.
2:      Sperm moving with a meandering, slow forward progression.
2+:   Sperm moving in a more direct slow forward course.
3:      Sperm moving in an almost straight line with moderate speed.
3+:   Sperm moving in a straight line with good speed.
4:      Sperm moving in a straight line with high speed.

Grade 3 is considered to indicate very good progression, and 2+ is the borderline between passable and poor motility. This system of grading is without question arbitrary and subjective; nevertheless, it gives excellent results when applied by an experienced observer.

On rare occasions a semen specimen will be seen in which all, or at least most, of the sperm cells appear to be motionless. In this case it is worthwhile to have the patient's blood tested for circulating sperm immobilizing antibodies.[19] (The details for performing the Isojima test for sperm immobilizing antibodies are discussed at the end of this chapter.)

Rare specimens will exhibit true necrospermia with absolutely no motility, and the eosin-nigrosin stain will be of diagnostic value in these cases (see later discussion).

When observed 2 or 3 hours after ejaculation at least 60 per cent of the sperm should have vigorous motility with good forward progression. When the specimen is kept in a glass or plastic container at room temperature, a slow but definite decline in the motility occurs, and at the end of 24 hours only a rare motile sperm cell is seen. It is not necessary to make repeated observations of the motility of the *in vitro* specimen because this is of no clinical significance. Such activity in the glass container over a period of hours cannot possibly be compared to the type of activity these cells will exhibit after they have been deposited in the vagina. As MacLeod points out, the seminal plasma is not a physiologic medium for preserving spermatozoa for a period of time longer than some minutes.[33, 34] Under the conditions of ejaculation in normal intercourse, the spermatozoa do not reach the main bulk of the seminal plasma in the urethra until the moment of ejaculation. There is no evidence that the seminal plasma in humans gets beyond the external os of the cervix. There is good evidence, however, in the immediate postcoital test[45] that the spermatozoa reach the cervical mucus within $1\frac{1}{2}$ minutes after ejaculation, and they cannot exist long in the vagina (in a mixture of seminal plasma and vaginal secretions) because of the high acidity of the vaginal secretions. Thus, it seems reasonably certain that the spermatozoa that eventually reach the vicinity of the ovum must pass into the cervical canal soon after ejaculation and therefore are quickly removed from the influence of the seminal plasma.

Poor sperm motility may occasionally be found in men with normal sperm counts after a long period of continence (10 days or more). This is probably due to the deterioration of the stored cells in the duct system; examination of a semen specimen from the same patient after a short period of abstinence may show a remarkable improvement in sperm motility.[36]

MORPHOLOGIC ASPECTS

Morphologic characteristics of the sperm cells should be given as much consideration as the cell count and motility. This can be accomplished only by smearing and staining the cells on a slide and performing a differential count on the stained smear. In the research laboratory, the Papanicolaou staining technique is an admirable method for staining the spermatozoa and showing the characteristics of the immature cells. However, this method is cumbersome for a physician who would like to determine the characteristics of the patient's semen in his own office laboratory. A practical method which allows rapid preparation of the slides for morphologic study involves the use of hematoxylin stain.

To prepare a smear, a drop of semen is placed near the end of an ordinary glass microscope slide and is spread from one side to the other using another slide, as is done in making a blood smear. The smear is then allowed to dry completely; it is not fixed with heat because this would distort some of the sperm and confuse the morphologic study. The air-dried smear is then fixed in 10 per cent formalin for 1 minute, rinsed in water, stained with Harris hematoxylin for 2 minutes, rinsed again in water, and allowed to dry. Should a counterstain be desired, the slide is placed after the second rinsing, in a solution of 0.1 per cent aqueous eosin for 5 to 10 seconds, rinsed in water, and allowed to air dry. The stain is not as elegant as that achieved with the Papanicolaou technique, but it is just as possible to classify the cells into the major categories by using this simple technique.

Research workers in the field of human seminal cytology have enumerated as many as 60 different morphologic types of mature spermatozoa,[12, 31, 32, 40, 51] but for practical purposes six major types may be used.[12] These types are oval or normal, large, small, tapering, duplicate, and amorphous cells.[31] These terms refer to the appearance of the head of the sperm, and the term amorphous is used to classify all mature cells that do not fall into the first five categories.

Immature cells of the germinal line may be exfoliated by the germinal epithelium, appearing thereafter in the ejaculum. These are sperm precursors, and when present, they should be included in the differential counts of the morphology. These immature or primitive sperm forms, such as spermatids or spermatocytes, should not be exfoliated or appear in the ejaculum under normal environmental conditions.

Difficulty in distinguishing between the white blood cells often seen in semen specimens and immature sperm forms may be a problem for the inexperienced observer. This can be overcome by using a fairly simple method: a 7-ml. blood sample is collected in a tube* containing 12 mg. disodium ethylenediaminetetraacetate (EDTA), the sample centrifuged, and the buffy coat containing the majority of the white blood cells removed. A normal semen specimen containing no immature forms is taken, and the buffy coat is added to this specimen. Smears are made and stained in the normal way, using hematoxylin. The inexperienced observer can then study the morphologic appearance of a semen specimen which contains a high percentage of white blood cells, and in this way learn to distinguish them from immature sperm forms.

Sperm morphology in man and animals is subject to great variation. One never sees a 100 per cent normal sample of human semen; that is, a certain percentage of deviations from the oval form regarded as normal is always present. The "80 per cent normal" entry in the records of the Margaret Sanger Research Bureau is infrequent, and the "90 per cent normal" designation is extremely rare. In other words, every semen sample contains at least 10 per cent abnormal sperm heads. The range of abnormal sperms may be seen in the photomicrographs presented in Figures 5-7 to 5-19. As noted, besides spermatozoa, many semen samples also contain structures such as sperm precursors in the spermatogenic line (spermatocytes and spermatids), as well as many kinds of cellular elements desquamated from the walls of the genital tract. Statistically, such cells are proportionately more numerous in semen specimens in which the sperm concentration (count per milliliter) is lowest.[17]

The purpose of these photomicrographs to provide the diagnostician with some idea of the diversity of pathology which he can expect to encounter in semen.

If there is much mucoid material in the semen which obscures good visualization of the spermatozoa, the slide can be rinsed with a few milliliters of Alevaire before it is stained, and this will eliminate the mucus.[1] However, this is not usually necessary.

In a fertile specimen, 60 per cent of at least 200 counted sperm should be normal (oval) in appearance. Sperm from one man tends to vary less in morphology than in count and motility, and may be compared to a fingerprint,[17, 30] except when some acute process (e.g., a viral infection, heat exposure) produces a temporary change. Occasional specimens of poor fertility are encountered in which the count and motility are excellent

Text continued on page 132

*Vacutainers (#3204Q) made by Beckton, Dickinson & Co., Rutherford, New Jersey 07073.

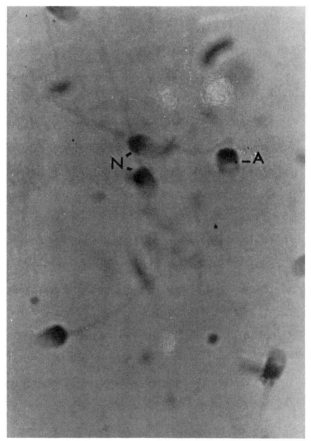

Figure 5-7.   Mostly normal (N) oval spermatozoa and one amorphous (A) shaped sperm.

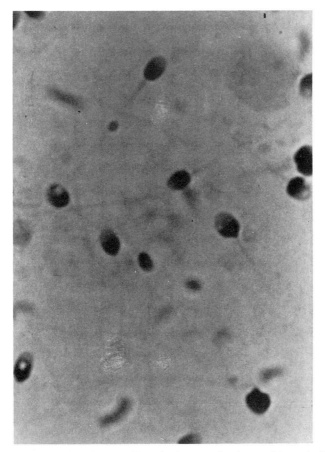

Figure 5-8. Normal oval sperm. Vacuoles in sperm heads are without significance.

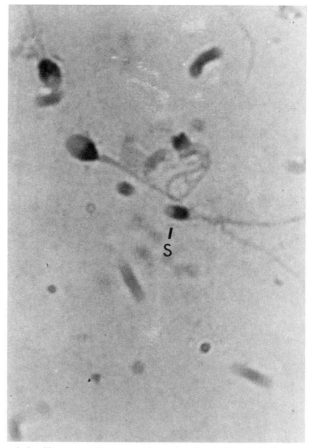

Figure 5–9. Two normal sperm and one small or microcephalic (S) sperm.

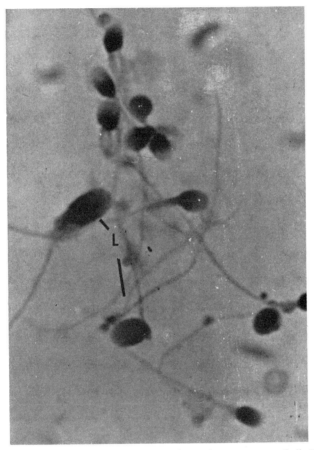

Figure 5–10.   Several normal spermatozoa and two giant or macrocephalic (L) sperm.

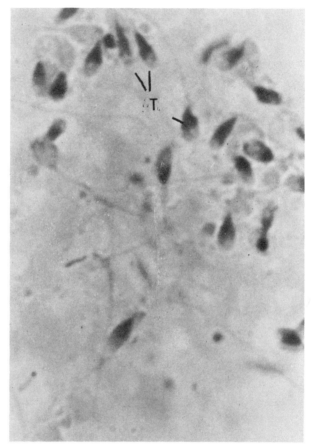

Figure 5–11.   A few normal sperm are present but most are of the tapering (T) type.

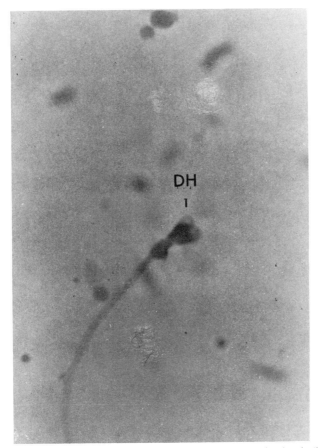

Figure 5–12. Duplicate-headed spermatozoa with two tapering heads (DH).

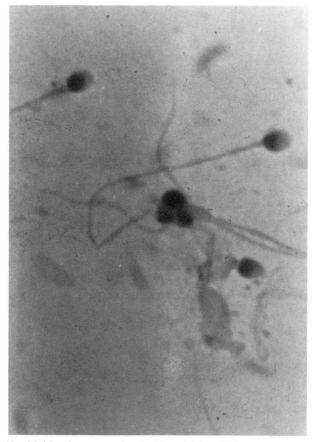

Figure 5–13. Multinuclear sperm head with multiple tails in center, surrounded by three normal oval sperm.

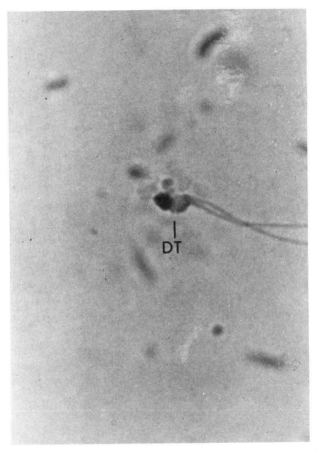

Figure 5-14. Duplicate-tailed sperm with small cytoplasmic droplet still in place (DT).

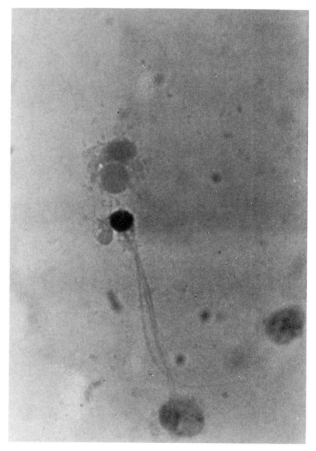

Figure 5–15. Multitailed sperm.

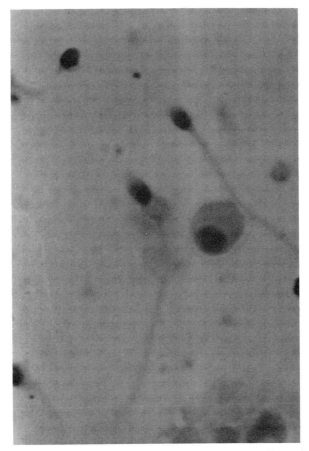

Figure 5–16. Normal oval sperm with huge cytoplasmic droplet still attached in neck and tail region.

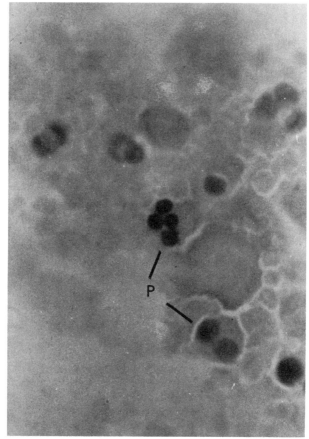

Figure 5–17. Primitive (P) cells. In center is a spermatid with four nuclei. At lower right is a secondary spermatocyte.

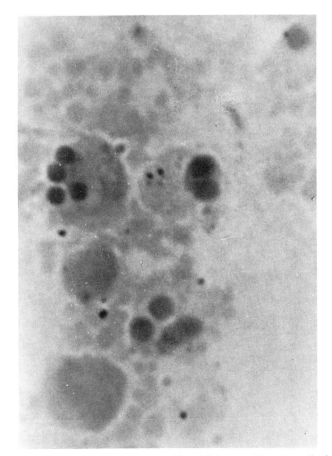

Figure 5–18.   Primitive cells. Two spermatids with four nuclei and a cell which has two nuclei, probably a secondary spermatocyte.

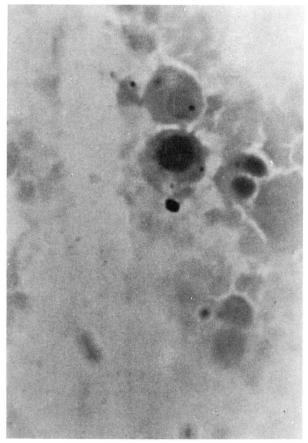

Figure 5-19. Various primitive cells. Cell with large nucleus is probably a primary spermatocyte.

and only the morphology is poor. Abnormal forms can have good motility, and great care should therefore be used to check sperm morphology.[35]

Sperm Morphology and Abnormalities of Pregnancy

MacLeod and Gold, in a series of papers analyzing the differences found in the semen quality of husbands in large fertile and infertile populations, have shown that it is not likely that sperm morphology is a factor in abnormalities of pregnancy or indeed, that semen quality in general plays a role in any type of pregnancy failure once the fact of conception has been well established.[35, 37] Other authors, including Hartman,[16] Bender,[6] Swyer,[47] and Joel,[20, 21] have also reached the conclusion that there is no relation between observed poor sperm morphology and accidents of pregnancy (miscarriage, ectopic pregnancy, or stillbirth). In fact, the semen quality of the husband in a large series of these cases is better than usual.[37] Recently, several papers have reported that low levels of deoxyribonucleic acid (DNA) in spermatozoa may be a cause of infertility or abortion,[22, 26, 27, 50] but this can not be detected in sperm morphology studies.

EOSIN-NIGROSIN STAIN

Distinguishing between live and dead spermatozoa is possible by using the eosin-nigrosin stain.[7, 52] Eosin in an aqueous solution cannot penetrate living cell membranes.

In this technique, stock solutions of 5 per cent eosin in distilled water and 10 per cent nigrosin in distilled water are kept separately. A drop of semen is placed on a glass slide. Next, a drop of eosin about double the size of the semen drop is placed on the slide, and finally a drop of nigrosin about twice the size of the eosin drop is deposited. By means of a glass rod, a brief but thorough mixing of the semen and the eosin droplet is effected, and when the mixture is homogeneous, the nigrosin drop is included in the final mixing process. After a few seconds of stirring the mixture is smeared in a thin layer onto a microscope slide, and the excess is discarded onto blotting paper under the slide. A thin smear is important if one is to attain the best differential results. The slide is then dried over a flame and is ready for microscopic examination, which is best done with the oil-immersion objective.

The difference between live and dead sperm cells can be clearly discerned, since those cells that are dead at the moment of mixing will have absorbed the eosin stain and show up with a distinct red color against the brownish-violet background. The living cells remain uncolored by the eosin.

This is an interesting technique, but it has limited practical application except in those discouraging cases in which the patient has no motile cells in the ejaculate and a diagnosis of true necrospermia can be made. It is of value as a research tool in perfecting techniques for freezing sperm, in which sperm survival must be evaluated and improved.[43]

OTHER TESTS ON SEMEN

pH

The pH of freshly ejaculated human semen is in the slightly alkaline range of 7.3 to 7.7, which is optimal for the survival of spermatozoa and does not vary to any significant extent in relation to semen quality.[39] On standing *in vitro*, there is an initial increase in pH as volatilization of the carbon dioxide from the semen renders it less acid, after which, there may be a decrease in pH due to metabolic accumulation of lactic acid, especially in specimens with high sperm concentrations.

FRUCTOSE

Seminal fructose is a product of the seminal vesicles, and its presence may be regarded as an index of androgenic stimulation. Fructose is present in all semen, with three notable exceptions: (1) in azoospermic males with congenital bilateral absence of the vas deferens. Semen from these men does not coagulate on ejaculation[2] because the seminal vesicles, which arise embryologically as an outbudding of the vasa deferentia, are also absent; (2) when both ejaculatory ducts are obstructed;[3] and (3) in an unusual form of retrograde ejaculation in which there is a scant initial outward ejaculate which is small in volume and contains no sperm.[24]

A simple test for the presence of seminal fructose may be performed as follows:[2] (1) Make up reagent by adding 50 mg. of powdered Resorcinol [USP] to 33 ml. of concentrated hydrochloric acid. Dilute to 100 ml. with distilled water. (2) Add 0.5 ml. of semen to 5 ml. of this reagent and bring to a boil. In the presence of fructose, an orange-red color will appear within 60 seconds after boiling. If fructose is absent, the solution will remain colorless (Fig. 5–20).

Every azoospermic specimen should be routinely tested for fructose by this simple method. By this means, any unsuspected case of sterility due to congenital absence of the vasa will be uncovered or confirmed without the necessity of scrotal exploration. If the reagent is stored under refrigeration in an amber bottle away from light, it will remain in good condition without discoloring for at least a year.

We have now examined over 150 azoospermic patients in whom the cause was congenital bilateral absence of the vas deferens. If the examiner can obtain a semen specimen from such an individual immediately after ejaculation (i.e., the specimen must be collected in the doctor's office) he will observe that the usual process of coagulation and liquefaction does not occur.[2] This is also explained by the concomitant absence of the seminal vesicles, which provide the substrate for normal coagulation. This simple test, a mere gross visual inspection, will enable an alert examiner to make a diagnosis even without examining the patient, but of course the semen specimen must be examined immediately (within 5 minutes) after ejaculation in order to do this, and the opportunity is lost when the specimen is collected at home and brought to the office for examination.

TESTS FOR IMMUNOLOGIC INCOMPATIBILITY AND INTERFERENCE

Although immunologic incompatibility and interference has been discussed in Chapter 4, the methodology necessary for the performance of three of the most utilized tests will be thoroughly discussed in this section.

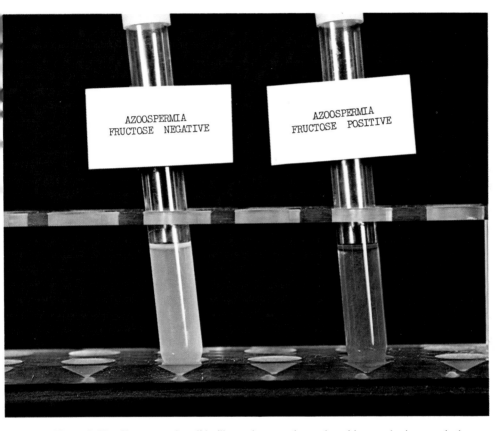

Figure 5–20.   Fructose color slide illustrating negative and positive results in a seminal fructose test of patients with azoospermia. If fructose is present, an orange-red color is obtained; if fructose is absent, the solution remains colorless. (From Amelar, R. D.: Infertility in Men. Philadelphia, F. A. Davis Co., 1966.)

THE KIBRICK TEST

The Kibrick sperm agglutination test (SPAT) was first described in 1952[25] and has recently been modified by Shulman.[44] Although this was the first method available that tested for the presence of circulating sperm-agglutinating antibodies, it did not become popular until recently owing to the complexity of methodology necessary to perform it.

A fresh semen specimen in which at least half of the sperm are motile with good forward progression and preferably number at least 80 million per milliliter is needed. Unfortunately, specimens with this count level are not always available, and on occasion one must settle for a count of as low as 60 million cells per milliliter. The sperm specimen is diluted with Baker's buffer[5] (glucose, 30.0 gm.; $Na_2HPO_4 \cdot 12H_2O$, 6.0 gm.; sodium chloride, 2.0 gm.; KH_2PO_4, 0.1 gm.; water to make 1000 ml.) to make a suspension of 40 million cells per milliliter. This diluted suspension of spermatozoa is diluted with an equal volume of 10 per cent gelatin made up with Baker's buffer and kept at 37° C.

The serum to be tested is inactivated at 56° C. for 30 minutes to destroy complement activity, which may otherwise cause a nonspecific agglutination or immobilization reaction to occur. The serum is then diluted with Baker's buffer 1:4, and 0.20 ml. of the diluted serum is added to 0.20 ml. of the sperm suspension in gelatin. The mixture is then gently agitated and transferred to small tubes with an inner diameter of 3 mm. and a length of about 3 cm.* These tubes are incubated at 37° C. and examined at intervals of 1 and 2 hours against a dark background and in front of a strong light. The presence of clumps and intervening clear fluid indicates a positive result. Sera that demonstrate positive agglutination at a dilution of 1:4 should be studied in serial dilution (e.g., 1:8, 1:16, 1:32 and so on).

Study of each serum sample should always utilize at least two semen specimens, and semen specimens that are free of any agglutination should be selected. Control sera, both positive and negative, must always be used when performing this test, not only for the usual technical reasons but also to evaluate the semen specimens employed. Should either the positive or negative controls produce an unexpected reaction, the results of all sera tested with that semen sample must be discarded.

If the semen sample to be tested has too low a sperm count (less than 60 million per ml.) or already exhibits significant sperm agglutination, donor semen specimens other than the husband's should be used, since the antigen appears to be species specific.

---

*These tubes are readily prepared from glass tubing cut into 3 cm. lengths with the end sealed in a flame, or they may be purchased from Arnel Products Company, 2701 Avenue U, Brooklyn, N.Y. 11229. A block of styrofoam makes a convenient rack for holding such tubes.

THE FRANKLIN-DUKES TEST

The Franklin-Dukes sperm agglutination test was first reported in 1964[10, 11] and was later adopted by Schwimmer and co-workers.[42] This method was one of the most extensively utilized sperm agglutination tests until recently, when it was demonstrated by Boettcher and co-workers that this test measures a nonimmunoglobulin, a beta-lipoprotein that can be influenced by varying hormone levels (see also Chapter 4).[8] The method described here has been slightly modified from that given in the original publications by Schulman[44] and is currently the method used in most laboratories.

A fresh semen specimen, in which at least 50 per cent of the sperm are motile with good forward progression, is diluted until it contains 50 million spermatozoa per milliliter. If the original concentration is less than 50 million per ml. the test cannot be done. All dilutions are made using Baker's buffer.[5] An aliquot of 0.05 ml. of the diluted semen specimen is then mixed with 0.50 ml. of a 1:4 dilution of the serum sample, which has been previously inactivated at 56° C. for 30 minutes. The mixture is then incubated at 37° C. After intervals of $\frac{1}{2}$, 1, 2, and 3 hours of incubation a drop is taken and examined under the microscope. The motile sperm cells are counted in each of 12 high-power fields, noting for every field the number of unclumped sperm cells, the number of cells in clumps, the number of clumps, and the type of clumping (head to head, tail to tail, etc.). The total number of cells clumped are divided by the total number of all motile sperm cells. If more than 20 per cent of the cells are clumped, the result is considered positive.

Should a serum sample be found to be positive, the exact titer may be established by serially diluting the sera (e.g., 1:8, 1:16, 1:32, and so on), adding the sperm cell suspension, and then reincubating.

As in the Kibrick sperm agglutination tests, positive and negative controls must be run in parallel with the test sera. As noted earlier, the test cannot be performed if the original sperm concentration in the specimen to be tested is less than 50 million per ml.

THE ISOJIMA TEST

The Isojima sperm immobilization test (SPIT) was first described in 1968.[19] It is a rather simple test that measures a complement-dependent antibody found in the sera of both men and women.

A fresh semen specimen having good sperm motility must be used. It is preferable that the sperm count be at least 80 million cells per milliliter, 50 per cent of them motile with a good forward progression. The semen specimen is diluted to 60 million cells per milliliter with Baker's buffer.[5]

The undiluted serum to be tested is inactivated at 56° C. for 30 minutes to remove any endogenous complement. The complement used in this test can be either fresh frozen guinea pig or rabbit complement. One must be warned about the use of lyophilized complement, since most diluents that are commercially available contain preservatives that will totally immobilize spermatozoa. The proportions to be used are as follows:

Test sera:
    Inactivated human sera   0.250 ml.
    Fresh human semen (60 million cells per ml.)   0.025 ml.
    Complement   0.050 ml.
Control:
    Inactivated human sera   0.250 ml.
    Fresh human semen (60 million cells per ml.)   0.025 ml.

The mixtures are placed in 10×75 mm. tubes, mixed, and incubated for 60 minutes at 37° C. The motility of the test serum is compared to that of the control for the same sera, and the sperm immobilization value (SIV) is determined by dividing the value of the control serum sperm motility by that of the test serum. If the SIV is found to be greater than 2, the test is considered positive. To obtain the titer of antibody present the positive sera may be serially diluted (e.g., 1:2, 1:4, 1:8, etc.) and the test redone using these dilutions.

A positive control sera should be used to ascertain that the semen specimen or the complement (or both) is not giving erroneous results. Additional negative controls should also be used as well as the mixture of the patient's sera and sperm minus complement, which acts as a negative control. Baker's buffer plus sperm and complement is a negative control, and normal, previously tested human sera plus complement and sperm is a second negative control.

Although the performance of the Kibrick, Franklin-Dukes and Isojima tests is beyond the capability of most physicians' office laboratories, the specific details of the techniques employed in these tests have been supplied for reference purposes for the interested reader.

REFERENCES

1. Amelar, R. D.: The use of Alevaire in the routine study of sperm morphology. Fertil. Steril., 7:346, 1956.
2. Amelar, R. D.: Coagulation, liquefaction and viscosity and human semen. J. Urol., 87:187, 1962.
3. Amelar, R. D., and Hotchkiss, R. S.: Congenital aplasia of the epididymides and vasa deferentia: effects on semen. Fertil. Steril., 14:44, 1963.
4. Amelar, R. D., Dubin, L., and Schoenfeld, C.: Semen analysis. Urology, 2:605, 1973.
5. Baker, J. R.: The spermicidal powers of chemical contraceptives. IV. More pure substances. J. Hyg., 32:171, 1932.
6. Bender, S.: The end-results in primary sterility. Brit. Med. J., 2:409, 1952.

7. Blom, E.: A one-minute live-dead sperm stain by means of eosin-nigrosin. Fertil. Steril., *1*:176, 1950.
8. Boettcher, B., Kay, D. J., Rümke, P., and Wright, L. E.: Human sera containing immunoglobulin and nonimmunoglobulin. Biol. Reprod., *5*:236, 1971.
9. Donne, A.: Cours de Microscopie. Paris, Balliere, 1844.
10. Franklin, R. R., and Dukes, C. D.: Antispermatozoal antibody and unexplained infertility. Amer. J. Obstet. Gynecol., *89*:6, 1964.
11. Franklin, R. R., and Dukes, C. D.: Further studies on sperm-agglutinating antibody and unexplained infertility. J.A.M.A., *190*:682, 1964.
12. Freund, M.: Standards for the rating of human sperm morphology. A cooperative study. Int. J. Fertil. (Suppl.), *11*:1, 1966.
13. Freund, M., and Carol, B.: Factors affecting haemocytometer counts of sperm concentration in human semen. J. Reprod. Fertil., *8*:149, 1964.
14. Gordon, J. A., Amelar, R. D., Dubin, L., and Tendler, M. D.: Infertility practice and orthodox Jewish law. Fertil. Steril., *26*:480, 1974.
15. Hartman, C. G.: Science and the Safe Period. Baltimore, The Williams and Wilkins Co., 1962.
16. Hartman, C. G.: Correlations among criteria of semen quality. Fertil. Steril., *16*:632, 1965.
17. Hartman, C. G., Schoenfeld, C., and Copeland, E.: Individualism in the picture of infertile men. Fertil. Steril., *15*:231, 1964.
18. Hotchkiss, R. S.: Fertility in Men. Philadelphia, J. B. Lippincott Company, 1944, pp. 113–115.
19. Isojima, S., Li, T. S., and Ashitaka, Y.: Immunologic analyses of sperm-immobilizing factor found in sera of women with unexplained sterility. Amer. J. Obstet. Gynecol., *101*:677, 1968.
20. Joel, C. A.: The role of spermatozoa in habitual abortion. Fertil. Steril., *6*:459, 1955.
21. Joel, C. A.: The spermatogenetic rebound phenomenon and its clinical significance. Fertil. Steril., *11*:384, 1960.
22. Joel, C. A.: New etiologic aspects of habitual abortion and infertility, with special reference to the male factor. Fertil. Steril., *17*:374, 1966.
23. Johnson, T. H.: A simple technique for direct semen examination. J. Urol., *89*:262, 1963.
24. Keiserman, W. M., Dubin, L., and Amelar, R. D.: A new type of retrograde ejaculation: Report of three cases. Fertil. Steril., *25*:1071, 1974.
25. Kibrick, S., Belding, D. L., and Merrill, B.: Methods for the detection of antibodies against mammalian spermatozoa. II. A gelatin agglutination test. Fertil. Steril., *3*:430, 1952.
26. Lenchtenberger, C.: The relation of DNA of sperm cells to fertility. J. Dairy Sci. (Suppl.), *43*:31, 1960.
27. Lenchtenberger, C., Weir, D. R., Schrader, F., and Mursames, L.: The DNA content of spermatozoa in repeated seminal fluid from fertile and infertile men. J. Lab. Clin. Med., *45*:851, 1955.
28. McLane, C. M.: Symposium of infertility. Clin. Obstet. Gynecol., *8*:11, 1965.
29. MacLeod, J.: Semen quality in one thousand men of known fertility and eight hundred cases of infertile marriage. Fertil. Steril., *2*:115, 1951.
30. MacLeod, J.: A possible factor in the etiology of human infertility: preliminary report. Fertil. Steril., *13*:29, 1962.
31. MacLeod, J.: Human seminal cytology as a sensitive indicator of the germinal epithelium. Int. J. Fertil., *9*:281, 1964.
32. MacLeod, J.: Human seminal cytology following the administration of certain antispermatogenic compounds. *In* Austin, C. R., and Perry, J. S. (eds.): Agents Affecting Fertility. Boston, Little, Brown and Co., 1965.
33. MacLeod, J.: The semen examination. Clin. Obstet. Gynecol., *8*:115–127, 1965.
34. MacLeod, J., and Gold, R. Z.: The male factor in fertility and infertility. III. An analysis of motile activity in the spermatozoa of 1000 fertile men and 1000 men in infertile marriage. Fertil. Steril., *2*:187, 1951.
35. MacLeod, J., and Gold, R. Z.: The male factor in fertility and infertility. IV. Sperm morphology in fertile and infertile marriage. Fertil. Steril., *2*:394, 1951.
36. MacLeod, J., and Gold, R. Z.: The male factor in fertility and infertility. V. Effect of continence on semen quality. Fertil. Steril., *3*:297, 1952.

37. MacLeod, J., and Gold, R. Z.: The male factor in fertility and infertility. IX. Semen quality in relation to accidents of pregnancy. Fertil. Steril., 8:36, 1957.
38. Macomber, D., and Sanders, M. B.: The spermatozoa count. N. Engl. J. Med., 200:981, 1929.
39. Mann, T.: The Biochemistry of Semen and of the Male Reproductive Tract. New York, John Wiley and Sons, 1964.
40. Moench, G. L., and Holt, H.: Sperm morphology in relation to fertility. Amer. J. Obstet. Gynec., 22:199, 1937.
41. Rehan, N. E., Sobrero, A. J., and Fertig, J. W.: The semen of fertile men. Statistical analysis of 1300 men. Fertil. Steril., 26:492, 1975.
42. Schwimmer, W. B., Ustay, K. A., and Behrman, S. J.: Sperm agglutinating antibodies and decreased fertility in prostitutes. Obstet. Gynecol., 30:192, 1967.
43. Sherman, J. K.: Synopsis of the use of frozen human semen since 1964: state of the art of human semen banking. Fertil. Steril., 24:397, 1973.
44. Shulman, S.: Immunologic barriers to fertility. Obstet. Gynec. Survey, 27:553, 1972.
45. Sims, J. M.: Clinical Notes on Uterine Surgery. New York, William Wood, 1866.
46. Sobrero, A. J., and MacLeod, J.: Immediate postcoital test. Fertil. Steril., 13:184, 1962.
47. Swyer, G. I. M.: Discussion of male infertility. Proc. R. Soc. Med., 46:835, 1953.
48. Syner, F. N., and Moghissi, K. S.: Purification and properties of a human seminal proteinase. Biochem. J., 126:1135, 1972.
49. Syner, F. N., Moghissi, K. S., and Yanez, J.: Isolation of a factor from normal human semen that accelerates dissolution of abnormal liquifying semen. Fertil. Steril., 26:1064, 1975.
50. Weir, D. R., and Lenchtenberger, C.: Low sperm DNA as a possible cause for otherwise unexplained human subfertility. Fertil. Steril., 8:373, 1957.
51. Williams, W. W.: Sterility. Springfield, Mass., Walter W. Williams, 1953.
52. Williams, W. W., and Pollak, O. J.: Study of sperm vitality with the aid of eosin-nigrosin stain. Fertil. Steril., 1:178, 1950.
53. Zorgniotti, A. W.: The spermatozoa count. A short history. Urology, 5:672, 1975.

Chapter 6

EXAMINING THE PATIENT

Richard D. Amelar, M.D.
Lawrence Dubin, M.D.

The man with a poor semen specimen must be investigated in an orderly fashion. The semen examination, while of great diagnostic value, is only one of several steps in evaluating the infertile male. Effective therapy is based upon treating the cause of the patient's impaired fertility.

A carefully performed history and physical examination are essential in the initial evaluation of the infertile male. We have found it helpful to use as a guide a printed form which can be filled in by the physician during the course of the examination. A copy of the survey summary form used in our practice is illustrated (Fig. 6–1). This is a 4-page form printed on both sides of a single folded sheet measuring 11 by 17 inches; it can be incorporated into the patient's chart.

THE HISTORY

In taking a thorough medical history of an infertile man, several general areas should be stressed and specific questions should be asked.

Text continued on page 146

MALE INFERTILITY SURVEY SUMMARY

Name _____ Wife's _____

Telephone - Home _____

Address _____ Office _____

Referred By: _____

Date: _____ Address: _____

	Age	Col.	Rel.	Education	Occupation	Former Occupation	Previous Marriages and Pregnancies
Husband							
Wife							

MARITAL HISTORY

Years Married _____ Liv. Child _____ Ages _____ Dead _____ Misc. _____ Ab (Ind.) (Spon.) _____ Ect. _____

Pregnanc. Total _____ Years of Pregnancies _____ Time to Conceive _____

Contraception (duration) _____ Methods: Condom _____ Rhythm _____ Pills _____ Diaph. _____ Other _____

Planning preg. (how long) _____

PRESENT HISTORY

General Health _____

Health Habits: _____ Tobacco _____ Alcohol _____

Present Complaints _____ Marihuana _____

Emotional Problems _____

FAMILY HISTORY

	Age	L	D	Cause	
Father					Sisters: s: _____ m. _____ ch. _____
Mother					Brothers: s: _____ m. _____ ch. _____

Familial Diseases _____

PAST HISTORY

Medical: Childhood _____ Mumps _____

_____ Other _____

Surgical: | Tonsillectomy _____ Appendectomy _____ Abdominal _____ Herniotomy _____

_____ Other _____

Remarks: _____ Allergies _____

_____ Medications _____

_____ Exposure to heat _____

_____ Military service _____

Signature _____

Figure 6-1. This 4-page survey form is used in our office practice for the evaluation of the infertile male.

Date

UROLOGICAL HISTORY

Testicular Descent   Varicocele

Infections

Treatments

SEXUAL HISTORY

Desire: Marked, Moderate, Slight, None   Frequency   Potency

Wife's Desires   Post-coital leakage

Marital Adjustment

Emotional Status

Personality

Previous Fertility Examinations and Treatments

Husband

Wife

Remarks:

Signature   M. D.

Figure 6–1 *Continued.*

SEE NEXT PAGE FOR
SEMEN ANALYSES

PHYSICAL EXAMINATION	date	LABORATORY REPORTS		
		TEST	DATE	RESULT
GENERAL APPEARANCE				
WEIGHT		URINE PROTEIN		
HEIGHT		URINE SUGAR		
SKIN		URINE MICROSCOPIC		
HEAD & NECK				
THYROID		PROSTATIC FLUID		
HEART				
PULSE		PROTEIN BOUND IODINE		
BLOOD PRESSURE		CHOLESTEROL		
LUNGS		PHOTOMOTOGRAM		
ABDOMEN		T_3 RESIN UPTAKE		
EXTREMITIES		T_4		
ENDOCRINOLOGICAL		17-KETOSTEROIDS		
HAIR DISTRIBUTION				
FAT DISTRIBUTION		PREGNANETRIOL		
GYNECOMASTIA				
ESCUTCHEON		17-OH		
PENIS				
SCROTUM		PITUITARY GONADOTROPHINS		
TESTES: RIGHT		FSH		
LEFT		LH		
EPIDIDYMIDES: RT		ESTROGENS		
LT		TESTOSTERONE		
VAS DEFERENS: RT				
LT		CHROMATIN PATTERN		
VARICOCELE RT		IMMUNOLOGICAL		husb. wife
LT		K¹BRICK SPAT		
PROSTATE				
SEMINAL VESICLES		ISOJIMA SPIT		
NEUROLOGICAL				
OTHER				
SUMMARY:				
DIRECTIONS:				

Figure 6–1 *Continued.*

SEMEN ANALYSES

DATE	Last Ejac. (Days)	Vol. ml.	Count (Millions Per ml.)	Count (Total)	Viscosity	MOTILITY			MORPHOLOGY							W.B.C.	FRUCTOSE
						Hrs	%	Grade	Normal Oval	Taper	Large	Small	Dupli-cate	Amorph	Primitive		

REMARKS

Figure 6–1 *Continued.*

OCCUPATION

Is there exposure to x-rays or radiation in the course of the patient's work? Does he work in a high-temperature environment (bakers, boiler makers, steam-fitters, laundry workers, for instance)? Does his job involve travel that may keep him away from home at the time of his wife's fertile periods? Does he work too hard or under undue tensions which leave him exhausted when he gets home? Does he take his job anxieties home with him?

GENERAL HEALTH

Has his health been adequate to have passed a medical examination for military service? If he was classified as 4F, what was the reason? Was he rejected for psychiatric reasons? Has he had any recent emotional shock?

What is the state of his present general health? Has his weight been steady or has he been gaining or losing weight? Has he been on any recent starvation diet to lose weight? Is he a diabetic, and if so, how is it controlled? Does he take any medications such as antihypertensive drugs or hormones such as thyroid or testosterone hormones or steroids that might upset his endocrine balance? Does he take vitamin pills? Does he have a well-balanced diet, avoiding in particular the recent diet fads in which protein, carbohydrate or fat is eliminated from the diet completely? Is there a satisfactory intake of vitamin foods, particularly the B-complex group? What is his intake of nicotine and alcohol? Does he use marihuana? Does he take any tranquilizing drugs or antidepressant agents? Is he on Dilantin therapy? What medications does he take, if any? Does he have any allergies?

Does he have any complaints that might suggest an endocrine disorder, such as tendency to gain weight easily out of proportion to his dietary intake, or a tendency to become easily fatigued and to feel sluggish? Is there an intolerance to temperature extremes?

Is there any history of severe childhood disease or any endocrine problem such as slow development or growth, marked obesity, or small genitalia for which endocrine therapy was administered? Has there been any severe kidney disorder which might be associated with uremia?

Has he had any kind of x-ray treatment (as for a skin condition or a tumor) or any unusually large number of diagnostic x-rays? (The patient often is unaware of what protective shielding measures, if any, were used to prevent damage to the seminiferous tubules.) Did he have mumps before or after puberty? If mumps occurred after puberty, was there any associated swelling of the testicles on one or both sides? Has he had any recent severe illnesses such as hepatitis that might have impaired his liver function? Has he had any febrile or viral illness within the past 3 months that might be reflected in a poor semen quality?

Has he had any operation for an inguinal hernia or a urologic problem such as a stone in the lower ureter which might have produced inadvertent damage to the spermatic blood vessels or the vas deferens?

Has there been any scrotal injury or infection such as epididymitis with swelling of the scrotal contents? Has he a history of scrotal pain suggesting intermittent testicular torsion? Has he been told that he has a varicocele? Have both testicles appeared to him to be equal in size? Has he ever had any urologic procedures that involved urethral instrumentation or prolonged indwelling of urethral catheters that might have produced scarring of the urethral ejaculatory ducts? Transurethral resection of urethral valves may inadvertently cause ejaculatory duct obstruction in the prostatic urethra. Has he had any nervous system disease or any surgery deep in the pelvis or retroperitoneum that might affect the neuromuscular mechanisms of ejaculation?

Does he take frequent hot baths that might expose his testicles to undesirably high temperatures? These should certainly be eliminated in favor of cooler baths or showers. It is a little known fact that strictly orthodox Jewish males as well as females may take daily hot baths (the Mikvah) as part of their religious practices.

Has the patient ever had any venereal infection, and if so, how was it treated? Has he had any sequelae such as urethral stricture or epididymitis? Has there been any prostatitis or nonspecific urethritis, and was it treated effectively?

Had both testicles descended into the scrotum at birth, or was there maldescent of one or both testicles? What measures were taken and at what age to bring the testicles into the scrotum, and were they successful? Even if correction of cryptorchism is carried out at about age 5 as suggested, the possibility of some surgical damage to the vas or blood supply at the time of the orchiopexy must be considered. The two-stage Torek procedure, in which the testicles are first buried in the subcutaneous tissue of the thighs and then released at a second stage, has been found more likely to compromise the vasculature of the testes than does the one-stage procedure.

SEXUAL HISTORY

Once the patient is assured of the physician's interest and sincerity, he will generally be willing to discuss intimate sexual relationships freely and without embarrassment. If fertility is a problem, it is important that coitus take place with a frequency that will make pregnancy possible. Are sex relations satisfactory with regard to the patient's ability to have orgasm with ejaculation while his penis is deeply within the vagina, or are there problems with erection, penetration, or premature ejaculation? Do the couple use coital lubricants such as petroleum jelly, Vaseline, K-Y jelly, Surgilube, or Lubrifax which are spermaticidal? A lubricant should not be necessary usually, but a small number of women with problems of infertility report inadequate vaginal lubrication during coitus and use commercial lubricants to remedy the problem. *Commercial vaginal lubricants should not be used by infertile couples.* If there is a need for added lubrication during coitus, saliva as a lubricant is both physiologic and readily available. Does the wife remain in bed after intercourse, or does she get up to go to the bathroom (or to douche)? Has the patient been experiencing difficulty having coitus on a schedule that may have been prescribed by a well-meaning doctor? Does he have frequent nocturnal emissions (usually associated with prolonged continence), or does he masturbate frequently? Does he have other frequent sexual outlets which may be cutting into his sexual desire for his wife or even impairing his semen quality?

Although frequent ejaculation (e.g., once daily) may have no clinically significant effect on the sperm count of a man who normally has high sperm production, such a practice can further reduce an already poor count. It is generally preferable to have sexual relations every other day rather than daily during the wife's fertile period if the sperm count is borderline. As already mentioned, sperm motility can be depressed by prolonged continence.

The orthodox Jew, who abstains from sexual contact until a full week after the last sign of menstrual flow, may be abstaining right through the fertile period and missing ovulation.

In dealing with patients with sexual dysfunction problems, it is most important to elicit a detailed sexual history. This is discussed in detail in Chapter 10.

It is often helpful to learn the results of previous fertility studies the patient may have had, although, since not all such studies are equally reliable, such information is sometimes confusing. The details of any previous therapy he may have received, including hormone pills and injections may also be helpful. For instance, if testosterone has recently been administered, it may be producing a spermatogenic depression. If the husband or wife has been married previously, information about the fertility of that marriage is again often helpful but occasionally confusing.

THE PHYSICAL EXAMINATION

The patient should be examined in the nude, so that the physician can obtain a general impression of possible endocrine stigmata from the body habitus, the amount and distribution of body hair, and the pattern of fat distribution. Such entities as Klinefelter's syndrome, Fröhlich's syndrome, severe hypothyroidism or hyperthyroidism, adrenogenital syndrome and eunuchism may be suspected from a first impression. Height, weight, any unusual length of extremities, and general nutritional status are noted.

A minimal neurologic examination for anosmia is important in the patient with hypogonadism to rule out Kallman's syndrome, a familial disease characterized by impaired olfactory acuity and isolated gonadotropin deficiency.[7, 8] Testing of visual fields is important in considering pituitary disorders. Patients with impotence should also be checked neurologically—a test of reflexes may suggest the presence of occult lumbar disc disease.[11]

The thyroid gland is carefully palpated. Cardiac irregularities may be detected on careful examination of the chest, and the breasts are carefully examined for gynecomastia. Abdominal palpation may reveal liver enlargement if present. Operative scars in the inguinal genital area are noted.

GENITALS

The examining room should not be cold—indeed, it should be warm—so that the scrotal dartos reflex will be relaxed, facilitating the examination of the genitalia. In this regard, we have found it helpful to place a warm lamp near the scrotum during the examination.

A complete examination of the genitalia should be made. The penis should not be unduly small. The urethral meatus should be in normal position and should not be stenotic. If hypospadias is present, it must be ascertained that the meatus is not displaced enough to make intravaginal deposition of semen difficult or impossible. In examining the scrotal contents, the position, size, and consistency of the testes are determined by gentle palpation. Because the seminiferous tubules account for 75 per cent of the testicular mass, the testes become soft and small when isolated damage to the seminiferous tubules has occurred. However, in the Sertoli cell-only syndrome of germinal cell aplasia, we have often found that the testes are normal in size and consistency. Normally the testes measure 4.6 cm. in length (range 3.6 to 5.5 cm.) and 2.6 cm. in width (range 2.1 to 3.2 cm.). Failure of descent of one or both testes may be discovered on physical examination. Polyorchidism is extremely rare and is not usually associated with normal spermatogenesis.[9]

A hydrocele as a cause of scrotal enlargement can be detected by transillumination in a darkened room. The epididymides can be palpated behind the testicles and any abnormality of size or consistency noted. Chronic epididymitis usually results in enlargement and induration of the structure, either in a localized segment such as the globus minor or in its entire extent. Spermatoceles are cysts arising usually from the head of the epididymis and can be diagnosed as encapsulated, transilluminating spherical structures above the testicle. The vas deferens should be palpated on both sides of the scrotum. It is often helpful to have the patient lie down on the examining table if this tubular structure cannot be palpated when the patient is erect. The frequency of congenital absence of the vas deferens, either unilaterally or bilaterally, is greater than one would expect from the relatively few reports in the literature. Indeed, 2 per cent of patients we have examined for infertility have been discovered to have bilateral congenital absence of the vas.[1,2] Calcification of the vas deferens is almost always associated with diabetes mellitus, and irregular beading may be a sign of tubercular involvement.

VARICOCELE

Most important, the patient should be examined for varicocele. Large and moderate sized varicoceles are easy to detect, but the diagnosis of a small varicocele requires some experience. A comparison of the size and bulk of the cord structures in the upright and recumbent positions is often helpful; a varicocele will usually disappear in the recumbent position. The varicocele can be made more pronounced in the erect position by having the patient perform the Valsalva maneuver.

With the patient standing upright before him, during the examination for varicocele the physician should seat himself on a comfortable stool and palpate the spermatic cords above the testes on both sides of the scrotum, using the thumbs and fingers of both hands to find and encircle these structures. The patient is then instructed to perform the Valsalva maneuver—he can be told to pinch his nostrils shut, close his mouth and strain as if he were going to move his bowels. This forced expiration with the glottis closed raises the intrathoracic pressure, impedes venous return to the heart, and thus increases venous pressure. With this maneuver, the small varicocele can be detected when present: the examiner will feel a backward impulse of the refluxing blood along the internal spermatic vein. The veins can then be emptied by finger pressure and the procedure repeated if necessary. Gentleness during this examination is to be stressed. An occasional patient may turn pale and, may even faint while being examined.

Varicoceles usually are present only on the left side but may be found bilaterally, as was the case in 15 per cent of our series (see Chapter 3), or rarely, only on the right side. Varicoceles may be significant whether small, moderate, or large in size.[4]

PROSTATE

The prostate gland is easily palpated by rectal digital examination unless the patient is markedly obese. The examiner will find the knee-chest position helpful for examination of the obese patient. The prostate should be symmetrical, of firm consistency, normal in size, and nontender to gentle palpation. Massage of the prostate is generally an uncomfortable procedure even to the normal male. Pain elicited by pressure to the prostate does not necessarily indicate that the gland is diseased. A prostate gland that is enlarged and boggy in consistency is often congested, infected, or both. Gentle massage of such a prostate may produce secretions which reveal numerous pus cells on microscope examination. The seminal vesicles normally are not palpable. If they are felt on rectal examination, an inflammatory abnormality or congenital cystic anomaly may be present.

Prostatitis may occasionally produce temporary impotence. Although many patients with prostatitis have no fertility problem, the presence of large numbers of *Escherichia coli* and related organisms is known to cause sperm agglutination in the infected ejaculum and to depress sperm motility *in vitro.*[13] Several recent reports have suggested that patients with infertility may have a high incidence of T-mycoplasma infections.[6] However, a recent prospective study has failed to demonstrate either a statistically significant increase in T-mycoplasma infections in barren couples or a significant effect on primary infertility,[5] as discussed in Chapter 4.

Prostatitis should be treated and cured if possible. It is best to avoid the use of nitrofurantoins for treatment because these drugs may cause damage to spermatocyte maturation, as demonstrated in a study of 36 men who were given therapeutic levels of the drug to combat urinary infection.[10] Irregular effects on the depression of spermatogenesis were seen in the sperm counts of 13 men and in the testicular biopsies of 7. It seems apparent from the literature that the depression of spermatogenesis by nitrofurantoins is dose-related and temporary.

Sperm cells are not usually found in the secretions expressed by prostatic massage in young men but are more common in older men who are having infrequent sexual relations.

SEMINAL VESICLES

The seminal vesicles are ordinarily not palpable unless they are congested or diseased. The rust-colored semen occasionally noticed by patients is most often due to congestive seminal vesiculitis. This is more likely to be noted when there is an irregular pattern of coital frequency, as in the case of a soldier sent to an isolated military base for a few months, then home on furlough for 2 weeks, and then back to his base.

URINALYSIS

A complete urinalysis is useful not only in detecting unsuspected renal disease or diabetes but also in suggesting the presence of lower urinary tract infections such as urethritis and cystitis. In the case of the patient who reports that he experiences orgasm but produces no detectable ejaculate, an immediate postorgasm urinalysis may enable the physician to make the diagnosis of retrograde ejaculation, in which large numbers of sperm will be found in the urinary sediment. It should be remembered that the acid pH of urine will immobilize sperm.

REFERENCES

1. Amelar, R. D., and Dubin, L.: Importance of careful palpation of vas deferens. Urology, 4:495, 1974.
2. Amelar, R. D., Dubin, L., and Schoenfeld, C.: Circulating sperm-agglutinating antibodies in azoospermic men with congenital bilateral absence of the vasa deferentia. Fertil. Steril., 26:228, 1975.
3. Bunge, R. G.: Some observations on the male ejaculate. Fertil. Steril., 21:639, 1970.
4. Dubin, L., and Amelar, R. D.: Varicocele size and results of varicocelectomy in selected subfertile men with varicocele. Fertil. Steril., 21:606, 1970.
5. DeLouvois, J., Harrison, R. F., Blades, M., Hurley, R., and Stanley, V. C.: Frequency of mycoplasma in fertile and infertile couples. Lancet, 1:1074, 1974.
6. Gnarpe, H., and Friberg, J.: T-mycoplasmas on spermatozoa and infertility. Nature, 245:97, 1973.
7. Hamilton, C. R., Jr., Henkin, R. I., Weir, G., and Kliman, B.: Olfactory status and response to clomiphene in male gonadotrophin deficiency. Ann. Intern. Med., 78:47, 1973.
8. Kallman, F. J., Schoenfeld, W. A., and Barrera, S. A.: The genetic aspects of primary eunuchoidism. Amer. J. Ment. Defic., 3:203, 1944.
9. Lazarus, B. A., and Tessler, A. N.: Polyorchidism with normal spermatogenesis. Urology, 3:615, 1974.
10. Nelson, W. O., and Bunge, R. G.: The effect of therapeutic dosages of nitrofurantoin (Furadantin) upon spermatogenesis in man. J. Urol., 77:275, 1957.
11. Shafer, N., and Rosenblum, J.: Occult lumbar disk causing impotency. N. Y. State J. Med., 69:2465, 1969.
12. Tagatz, G. E., Okagaki, T., and Sciarra, J.: Effect of vaginal lubricants on sperm motility and viability in vitro. Amer. J. Obstet. Gynecol., 113:88, 1972.
13. Teague, N. S., Boyarsky, S., and Glenn, J. F.: Interference of human spermatozoan motility by *Escherichia coli.* Fertil. Steril., 22:281, 1971.

Chapter 7

ENDOCRINE EVALUATION OF THE INFERTILE MALE

PATRICK C. WALSH, M.D.

In Chapter 2 the various endocrine disorders associated with male infertility were classified into three broad categories: abnormalities of hypothalamic function, abnormalities of pituitary function, and abnormalities of testicular function. With the widespread availability of reliable immunoassays for the measurement of serum LH, FSH, and testosterone, it is possible for the clinician to determine accurately whether gonadotropin deficiency or primary testicular failure is the cause of disordered testicular function. In rare instances when the clinical findings suggest an abnormality of thyroid or adrenal function, additional endocrine tests may identify the presence of one of these unusual disorders. This chapter discusses the methodology and interpretation of the laboratory tests used in the evaluation of endocrine function in infertile men.

EVALUATION OF THE HYPOTHALAMIC-PITUITARY-TESTICULAR AXIS

The measurement of serum levels of LH, FSH, and testosterone can be most helpful in the evaluation of the infertile male. Because of episodic fluctuations of serum LH and testosterone levels, the range of normal values is quite broad. Over a 24-hour period there are approximately 9 to 14 peaks of LH, and changes in the blood level may increase ninefold from nadir to peak.[3, 13, 18] Alterations in testosterone levels are somewhat less, ranging from an increase of less than twofold to greater than threefold.[11] For this reason, under certain circumstances it may be necessary to collect serial samples; for example, multiple sampling is most useful in circumstances where LH levels are borderline low or equivocal. However, in most patients, single samples are satisfactory for routine screening. Serum levels of FSH show little fluctuation because the metabolic clearance of FSH is slower than the clearance of LH, thereby producing a longer survival of FSH in the plasma.[12] Although in most cases the measurements of LH and FSH are precise, it is important to recognize that in patients with gonadotropin deficiency, there is always some measurable gonadotropin in the plasma. Consequently, for an adequate interpretation of gonadotropin levels, it is essential to know the level of testosterone in the plasma.

In patients with symptoms and signs of androgen deficiency who have low plasma testosterone levels, the measurement of serum LH and FSH can differentiate hypogonadotropic eunuchoidism from primary testicular disease. If plasma gonadotropin levels are elevated, then the patient has primary testicular disease. If plasma gonadotropin levels are low or borderline normal, then a diagnosis of hypogonadotropic eunuchoidism can be made. Occasionally, if the results are equivocal the clomiphene stimulation test may be useful.[14] Clomiphene is a nonsteroidal compound with antiestrogenic activity. Following treatment with clomiphene, the negative feedback effect of testicular steroids on the pituitary is blocked; consequently in the normal patient there is an increase in serum LH and FSH levels. In patients with borderline low gonadotropin levels, it is possible to determine whether these levels can be stimulated by administering clomiphene, 50 mg. twice a day for 7 days. The minimum normal response during clomiphene administration has been defined as an increase over control levels of 30 per cent for LH and 22 per cent for FSH.[14] To determine whether the cause of hypogonadotropism is due to a defect in the hypothalamus or pituitary, treatment with GnRH (100 μg subcutaneously) has been advised. Unfortunately, this test does not reliably distinguish between these two disorders because in patients with hypothalamic deficiency, the pituitary gonadotropins must be exposed to GnRH for prolonged periods before a normal adult response occurs.[10]

More commonly, patients who present with primary infertility have normal Leydig cell function with normal plasma testosterone and LH levels.[17] In these patients, the measurement of plasma FSH can be most helpful. Although castration results in a marked increase in plasma LH and FSH, isolated damage to the seminiferous tubules leaving Leydig cell function intact causes an isolated increase in serum FSH levels. A number of studies have demonstrated that in patients with infertility, elevated serum FSH levels are most frequently found in association with severe damage to the seminiferous tubules.[2, 6, 9, 15, 19] These elevated levels of FSH are almost always associated with a reduction in all germinal elements, including spermatogonia. Consequently, in the patient with small testes and severe oligospermia or azoospermia, the presence of elevated serum FSH levels is conclusive evidence of severe tubular damage. In these patients, a testicular biopsy is generally not necessary. Conversely, in the patient with azoospermia due to ductal obstruction, plasma FSH levels are normal. Finally, in patients with hyalinization of the seminiferous tubules and Leydig cell dysfunction (e.g., Klinefelter's syndrome), serum LH and FSH are both elevated. These findings are depicted diagramatically in Table 7–1.

Table 7–1 SERUM GONADOTROPIN AND TESTOSTERONE LEVELS IN INFERTILE MEN

	LH	*FSH*	*T*
Idiopathic oligospermia	←→	←→	←→
Maturation arrest	←→	←→	←→
Ductal obstruction	←→	←→	←→
Gonadotropin deficiency	↓ →	↓ →	↓
Sertoli cell only	←→	↑	←→
Seminiferous tubule hyalinization	↑	↑	↓ →

←→ = Normal, ↑ = Elevated, ↓ = Low

EVALUATION OF CHROMOSOMAL ABNORMALITIES

A quick and often helpful laboratory test used to screen patients for the presence of sex chromosomal abnormalities is the examination of buccal mucosal cells for the presence of chromatin clumps on the nuclear membrane—the Barr body. The Barr body, which represents the second X chromosome, is found in 20 per cent or more of the nuclei of normal females and in less than 2 per cent of cells from normal males. This test is useful in detecting the presence of more than one X chromosome. If the buccal mucosal cells are stained with quinacrine or its mustard derivative and examined by fluorescent microscopic techniques, the Y chromosome can also be identified. This method, which was described by Caspersson and associates, provides a rapid means of identifying the presence of a Y chromosome.[4] Consequently, the presence of additional X and Y chromosomes can be identified from a buccal mucosal preparation.

The more direct means of determining the human chromosomal complement involves the culture of peripheral blood leukocytes in media containing a mitogenic agent (phytohemagglutinin), which induces the lymphocytes to divide after a 3-day period of exposure at 30° C. Colchicine, which arrests mitosis at metaphase, is added to the cells, which are then harvested, put on slides, and stained. The chromosomes of a number of cells in metaphase are then counted to establish the number per cell. This technique is valuable in determining the exact chromosomal complement and the presence of mosaicism, autosomal abnormalities, and structural chromosomal alterations. However, to determine mosaicism accurately, the study of multiple tissues may be necessary. Finally, in the future, the measurement of the H–Y antigen may be most helpful in detecting the presence of the testis-determining factor in selected patients.[20]

EVALUATION OF THYROID FUNCTION

Thyroid dysfunction is such a rare cause of male infertility that routine screening of infertile men for abnormalities of thyroid function should be discouraged. Only those patients with clinical findings suggestive of hyperthyroidism or myxedema should be studied. The measurement of thyroid hormones in the serum represents the simplest, most readily available, and probably the most useful laboratory test for thyroid function. However, because both thyroxin (T_4) and tri-iodothyronine (T_3) bind to plasma proteins, changes in the hormone concentration in the blood may reflect a primary alteration in hormone binding rather than hormone supply.[16] Consequently, the physician is concerned mostly with the concentration of the two "free" thyroid hormones. Because there is no direct method for determining these concentrations, several measurements must be used to arrive at an estimate. Total serum T_4 levels can be assayed by nonchemical competitive protein-binding methods. The normal value of serum T_4 by this technique varies between 4 and 11 μg per 100 ml. Circulating T_3 levels, measured by radioimmunoassay, range from 100 to 200 ng. per 100 ml. The concentration of circulating T_4 reliably reflects T_4 secretion when the binding capacity of the transport proteins is normal, but this is not true when there are pronounced alterations in binding capacity.[16] When circulating thyroid-binding globulin (TBG) is increased, the serum T_4 is generally abnormally high. Consequently, to interpret serum T_4 levels adequately, an estimation of the free T_4 or TBG capacity is necessary. By adding a tracer quantity of labeled hormone to serum containing an insoluble material such as charcoal and measuring the fraction of the hormone retained in the insoluble phase, the "T_3 uptake" or resin uptake can be determined; this provides an inverse measurement of the serum protein binding capacity.[16] Since the enhanced secretion of thyroid hormone in hyperthyroidism leads to a greater than normal degree of saturation of the binding protein with T_4, the resin uptake tends to be high in hyperthyroidism. In hypothyroidism, in which thyroid hormone secretion is low, the serum proteins are undersaturated and the resin uptake is low. Although neither the resin uptake nor the serum T_4 is an invariably reliable index of thyroid status, a combination of these two tests may be very helpful. In hypothyroidism, serum T_3 and T_4 are low, and the resin uptake is low. In hyperthyroidism, serum T_3 and T_4 levels are higher than normal and the resin uptake is increased. In addition, patients in whom hyperthyroidism is a cause of infertility frequently have elevated serum levels of testosterone and LH.[5]

EVALUATION OF ADRENAL FUNCTION

Because well-documented cases of adrenal dysfunction giving rise to male infertility are very rare, only those patients with clinical findings suggestive of congenital adrenal hyperplasia should be studied. Some authors have suggested that a mild form of congenital adrenal hyperplasia, possibly acquired, may play a significant role in the pathogenesis of male infertility. However, the existence of this disorder is highly questionable. In the past, the diagnosis of this disorder has been based on the finding of elevated 17-ketosteroid levels in the urine,[1] but elevations of 17-ketosteroids may be nonspecific, and better documentation is necessary before one can make this diagnosis with confidence. In the 21-hydroxylase deficiency, elevated serum levels of 17-hydroxyprogesterone and increased urinary pregnanetriol should be present. In the 11-hydroxylase deficiency, there should be elevated serum levels of 11-deoxycortisol and increased urinary excretion of tetrahydro S.

REFERENCES

1. Amelar, R. D., and Dubin, L.: Male infertility. Current diagnosis and treatment. Urology, *1*:1, 1973.
2. Baker, H. W. G. *et al.*: Testicular control of follicle-stimulating hormone secretion. Recent Progr. Horm. Res., *32*:429, 1976.
3. Boyar, R., Perlow, M., Hellman, L., Kapen, S., and Weitzman, E.: Twenty-four hour pattern of luteinizing hormone secretion in normal men with sleep stage recording. J. Clin. Endocrinol. Metab., *35*:73, 1972.
4. Caspersson, T., Hulten, M., Jonasson, J., Lindsten, J., Therkelsen, A., and Zech, L.: Translocations causing non-fluorescent Y chromosomes in human XO/XY mosaics. Hereditas, *68*:317, 1971.
5. Clyde, H. R., Walsh, P. C., and English, R. W.: Elevated plasma testosterone and gonadotropin levels in infertile males with hyperthyroidism. Fertil. Steril., *27*:662, 1976.
6. de Kretser, D. M., Burger, H. G., and Hudson, B.: The relationship between germinal cells and serum FSH levels in males with infertility. J. Clin. Endocrinol. Metab., *38*:787, 1974.
7. Franchimont, P., Millet, D., Vendrely, E., Letawe, J., Legros, J. J., and Netter, A.: Relationship between spermatogenesis and serum gonadotropin levels in azoospermia and oligospermia. J. Clin. Endocrinol. Metab., *34*:1003, 1972.
8. Hunter, W. M., Edmond, P., Watson, G. S., and McLean, N.: Plasma LH and FSH levels in subfertile men. J. Clin. Endocrinol. Metab., *39*:740, 1974.
9. Leonard, J. M., Leach, R. B., Couture, M., and Paulsen, C. A.: Plasma and urinary follicle-stimulating hormone levels in oligospermia. J. Clin. Endocrinol. Metab., *34*:209, 1972.
10. Mortimer, C. H., Besser, G. M., McNeilly, A. S., *et al.*: Luteinizing hormone and follicle-stimulating hormone releasing hormone test in patients with hypothalamic-pituitary-gonadal dysfunction. Brit. Med. J., *4*:23, 1973.

11. Naftolin, F., Judd, H. L., and Yen, S. S. C.: Pulsatile patterns of gonadotropins and testosterone in man: the effects of clomiphene with and without testosterone. J. Clin. Endocrinol. Metab., *36*:285, 1973.

12. Naftolin, F., Yen, S. S. C., and Tsai, C. C.: Rapid cycling of plasma gonadotropins in normal men as demonstrated by frequent sampling. Nature [New Biol.] *236*:92, 1972.

13. Nankin, H. R., and Troen, P.: Repetitive luteinizing hormone elevations in serum of normal men. J. Clin. Endocrinol. Metab., *33*:558, 1971.

14. Paulsen, C. A.: The testes. *In* Williams, R. H. (ed.): Textbook of Endocrinology, 5th ed. Philadelphia, W. B. Saunders Co., 1974, p. 323–367.

15. Rosen, S. W., and Weintraub, B. D.: Monotropic increase of serum FSH correlated with low sperm count in young men with idiopathic oligospermia and azoospermia. J. Clin. Endocrinol. Metab., *32*:410, 1971.

16. Rosenberg, I. N.: Evaluation of thyroid function. N Engl. J. Med., *286*:924, 1972.

17. Ruder, H. J., Lorianx, D. L., Sherins, R. J., and Lipsett, M. B.: Leydig cell function in men with disorders of spermatogenesis. J. Clin. Endocrinol. Metab., *38*:244, 1974.

18. Santen, R. J., and Bardin, C. W.: Episodic luteinizing hormone secretion in man. Pulse analysis, clinical interpretation, physiologic mechanisms. J. Clin. Invest., *52*:2617, 1973.

19. Van Thiel, D. H., Sherins, R. J., Myers, G. H., Jr., and De Vita, V. T., Jr.: Evidence for a specific seminiferous tubular factor affecting follicle-stimulating hormone secretion in man. J. Clin. Invest., *51*:1009, 1972.

20. Wachtel, S. S., Koo, G. C., Breg, W. R. *et al.*: Serologic detection of a Y-linked gene in XX males and XX true hermaphrodites. N. Engl. J. Med., *295*:750, 1976.

Chapter 8

TESTICULAR BIOPSY

LAWRENCE DUBIN, M.D.
RICHARD D. AMELAR, M.D.

The role of testicular biopsy in the diagnosis and treatment of male infertility has certainly been less prominent in recent years.[10] Adequate staining and study of cellular morphology in the ejaculate often yield more information than biopsy of the testicle itself in oligospermic males. We usually reserve biopsy for differentiation of primary testicular failure from obstruction of the vas or epididymis in azoospermic men.

Indeed, some recent studies have shown marked sperm suppression following testicular biopsy. Rowley et al.[19] studied 100 normal volunteers who had testicular biopsies. Thirty-nine patients exhibited significant drops in sperm counts starting 3 weeks after biopsy. Recovery of previous sperm levels was not achieved for 10 to 18 weeks. Another problem may arise if sperm are spilled at the time of biopsy, resulting in subsequent antibody formation. This, however, has not been definitely proved at present.

Nevertheless, other investigators feel that testicular biopsy offers a

159

guide to diagnosis, prognosis, and choice of treatment in oligospermic as well as azoospermic men.[5, 11] Certainly a full knowledge of the technique and interpretation of testicular biopsy is important to those interested in male infertility.

GENERAL TECHNICAL CONSIDERATIONS

The technique of biopsy of the testes is more important than that in other areas of the body. Testicular tissue is fragile, and needle biopsy is impossible without derangment of testicular architecture.

Fixation of the specimen is probably the one procedure that is most often poorly performed. Formalin and formaldehyde solutions completely destroy the testicular ultrastructure and make the biopsy impossible to interpret. When formalin is used for fixation, the tubules will shrink, the germinal cells will be distorted, the nuclei will become pyknotic, and differentiation between the stages of maturation is impossible. Biopsy specimens may be fixed in Zenker's, Bouin's, or Carnoy's solution, and it is the surgeon's responsibility to see that the tissue is placed in the proper fixative.

Biopsies should be performed bilaterally because of the occasional difference of pathology on the two sides. Some physicians perform vasography at the same time. This is to be severely condemned because vasography in itself is traumatic and may cause irreparable obstruction of the vas. If any sperm at all are present in the ejaculate obstruction of both vasa is certainly impossible, and the procedure of vasography is totally unnecessary. If the patient is azoospermic, the procedure should be done if necessary at the time of epididymovasostomy or vasovasostomy when all structures are exposed and reparative surgery can be done immediately. It is, therefore, not necessary to explore the scrotum during the biopsy procedure.

Testicular biopsies should be performed in an operating room under strict aseptic conditions. Local or general anesthesia may be used, although we prefer general anesthesia since there is less discomfort and the procedure is of short duration. Under local anesthesia, the patient may feel momentary pain referred to the lower abdomen when the tunica albuginea is incised or sutured. If he is warned of this impending discomfort in advance, his apprehension will be allayed.

As a precaution, it is generally preferable to use a general anesthetic rather than a local one in patients who have scrotal inflammation with orchitis, because of the dense adhesions that may distort the landmarks around the testicle. A general anesthetic is also preferred if the patient has a large varicocele because there are usually large veins over the anterior surface of the testicle within the tunica vaginalis; these must be exposed and avoided to prevent troublesome bleeding.

SURGICAL PROCEDURE

The scrotal area is shaved and scrubbed and prepared with an antiseptic such as Betadine. The testicle is held in position with the scrotal skin pulled tense over its anterior aspect. Great care must be used to ascertain that the epididymis is in its proper posterior location before any incision is made. Indeed, mistaken incision into the epididymis will cause epididymal obstruction and sterility, since the epididymis is a solitary tube 22 feet long with a convoluted anatomic configuration.

A transverse incision 1 to 2 cm. long is made, avoiding the large vessels in the skin. It is gently carried down to the depth of the tunica vaginalis. The tunica vaginalis is then incised in the same direction. When this structure is incised a small amount of clear fluid is characteristically released, making it simple to identify and pick up the edges of the tunica vaginalis with hemostats. The incision in the tunica vaginalis is then extended to the length of the scrotal skin incision. Excellent exposure of the midportion of the anterior surface of the underlying testis can be obtained, using hemostats or small vein retractors (Fig. 8–1).

A 4–0 chromic atraumatic fixation suture is placed at the upper pole of the incision into the tunica albuginea, and the tunica albuginea is incised transversely to avoid cutting across small superficial branches of the spermatic artery which run in a transverse direction from the posterior to the anterior portions of the testicle. A small bit of testicular stroma will protrude, and a 2 mm. square portion is cut off with a small sharp pair of scissors.

Gentle pressure may be applied to the sides of the testicle to assist in forcing the testicular tissue to protrude. After this tissue is removed for biopsy, it is immediately placed with minimal handling in a labeled jar containing Bouin's, Zenker's, or Carnoy's solution. The edges of the incision in the tunica albuginea are then approximated with 3–0 or 4–0 atraumatic chromic catgut suture material. The tunica vaginalis is closed with 3–0 or 4–0 chromic catgut, and the skin is then approximated with 3–0 or 4–0 plain catgut sutures.

After the same procedure has been repeated on the other side, a small Telfa dressing and a scrotal suspensory are applied. After a local anesthetic, the patient may be discharged the same day; after a general anesthetic he may leave the following morning. The dressings are removed in 2 days and he is allowed to take showers. The catgut skin sutures will absorb in about 1 week.

INTERPRETATION OF BIOPSY

The testes have two functional components, the tubules and the interstitial cells. The tubules are lined by seminiferous epithelium. All the cells

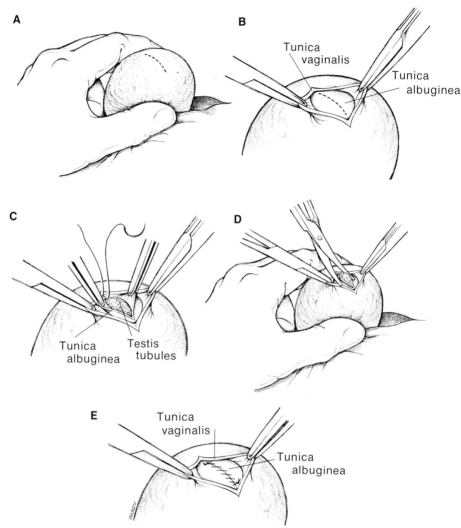

Figure 8-1. Method of testicular biopsy. *A.* The testicle is held in position with the scrotal skin pulled tense over its anterior aspect. A transverse incision 1 to 2 cm. in length is made and is carried down to the tunica vaginalis. *B.* The tunica vaginalis is then incised in the same direction, exposing the tunica albuginea. The edges of the tunica vaginalis are grasped with hemostats. *C.* A 4–0 atraumatic chromic fixation suture is placed at the upper pole of the incision into the tunica albuginea, and the tunica albuginea is incised transversely. *D.* A small bit of testicular stroma will extrude, and a 2 mm. square portion is cut off with a small sharp pair of scissors. *E.* The tunica albuginea is closed with 4–0 chromic atraumatic sutures.

of the epithelium except the Sertoli cells are involved in spermatogenesis. The interstitial cells are usually clumps of endocrine cells located in the connective tissue supporting the tubules.

The testes are incompletely partitioned by septa originating in the thick fibrous testicular capsule known as the tunica albuginea. In the hilar area of the testes the capsule is more dense and is traversed by the 9 to 15 epithelial ducts of the rete testis. It must be remembered that the spermatozoa in the testis, even in the rete, are not capable of fertilizing ova, and that maturation is completed in the epididymis and vas deferens.

HISTOLOGY

As stated earlier, there are six stages in the development of mature spermatozoa.[13] In histologic sections, the secondary spermatocytes are rarely seen. A cross-section of any normal seminiferous tubule reveals four or five distinct generations of germ cells. The younger generation cells are at the basement membrane, and the more differentiated cells approach the lumen of the tubule. This growth pattern has a wavelike cycle with intermingling of different stages in close approximation. Thus, one or two generations of cells tend to remain grouped, and these cell groupings remain intact throughout the successive cycles. Thus, any single cross-section of the tubule does not always reveal all generations of spermatogenesis. In addition to the admixture of various generations of cells that appear to disrupt the smooth flow of maturation from spermatogonia to spermatozoa, the cells of another adjacent wave intermingle with these at the border of the cellular association. This seeming dissociation is normal. The tubules rest on a delicate anuclear basement membrane which in turn rests upon a connective tissue layer, the tunica propria.

The round tubules are separated from each other by a small amount of connective tissue containing, in addition to blood vessels, a few lymphocytes, plasma cells, and clumps of interstitial cells. The interstitial cells are large, more than 20 microns in diameter. The nuclei are usually oval or spherical, and some are binucleated. The cytoplasm contains lipoid droplets and a perinuclear granular zone. Some of the cells contain pigment which is neither melanin nor a blood pigment derivative; the precise nature and significance of this pigment have yet to be established. The interstitial cells constitute a well-vascularized diffuse type of endocrine gland which develops from a mesenchymal stroma rather than from an epithelial surface as do other endocrine structures.

The Sertoli cells are believed to nourish the germ cells. They are large cells with large pale nuclei, polymorphous in shape. The abundant cytoplasm extends from the periphery of the tubule to the lumen, stretching through the layers of developing germ cells. The mature spermatozoa are seen attached to and surrounding the Sertoli cells prior to their release.

The normal testis has tubules that are surprisingly uniform in size. The tubular lumina are easily seen. In the normal, nontraumatized, well-fixed specimen, the lumina contain relatively few mature cell forms.

Testicular abnormalities may be multiple, and exact classification is difficult. Empathy between the pathologist and the clinician is necessary in order to avoid a wreck on semantic rocks. Much of the following material is taken from Dr. Warren O. Nelson's classic work in this field.[16]

Commonly, one of five histologic patterns may be found, alone or in combination, in testicular biopsies.[2, 3, 9, 16]

Normal Testicles. This pattern may be encountered in azoospermic patients in whom there is an obstruction of the conducting passages, or in whom there is a congenital absence of the epididymis or vas deferens (Fig. 8–2). Occasionally, biopsies from men with oligospermia show a surprisingly normal appearance, which is unexplained.

Spermatogenic Maturation Arrest. Commonly encountered in oligospermia, this is a condition in which the spermatogenic process fails to progress beyond one of the early stages (Fig. 8–3). The testes are usually somewhat reduced in size and the tubules reflect this reduction. As a rule the spermatogonia are normal in numbers until the primary spermatocytes are formed, when the process seems to break down. The number of primary spermatocytes is therefore increased, but few or no advanced stages of maturation are seen. The increased development may occur at the secondary spermatocyte stage, as in cases when the effect of heat damage on the testes has been noted. Less frequently, maturation may proceed to the spermatid stage and be arrested there. In any event, the result is the same—very few or no sperm are produced. The arrested cells, whatever the stage of their development, undergo fragmentation and slough into the tubular lumina. The exact cause of spermatogenic maturation arrest is frequently indeterminable, but one or more defects in the mechanisms of chromosomal synapse and division may be responsible. Careful study of the abortive attempts of primary spermatocytes to carry out the complicated process of the first maturation division strongly suggests a serious disturbance in chromosomal function. Other possible causes of spermatogenic maturation arrest are failure of the Sertoli cells to provide the nutritive environment necessary for spermatogenesis, and defective action of the gonadotropic hormones.

Peritubular Fibrosis. This is an entity of unknown cause in which there is a progressive depletion of the nourishment of the spermatogenic tubules with consequent atrophy and hyalinization (Fig. 8–4). Mild early cases are probably not clinically significant, but more advanced conditions are associated with correspondingly greater seminal deficiency. In many cases, the process of fibrosis is progressive and eventually may be expected to involve larger numbers of tubules, as shown by serial biopsies.[17] Although peritubular fibrosis has commonly been regarded as irreversible, it has been shown by Heller *et al.*[14] that severe fibrosis occurring in the testes of men receiving testosterone propionate disappeared after cessation of treatment. Further study may reveal the existence of different types of peritubular fibrosis, but in most cases it appears to progress until all the germ cells are eliminated and the tubules are completely sclerosed. This condition has been seen in patients with histories of testicular trauma, severe infections such

Text continued on page 169

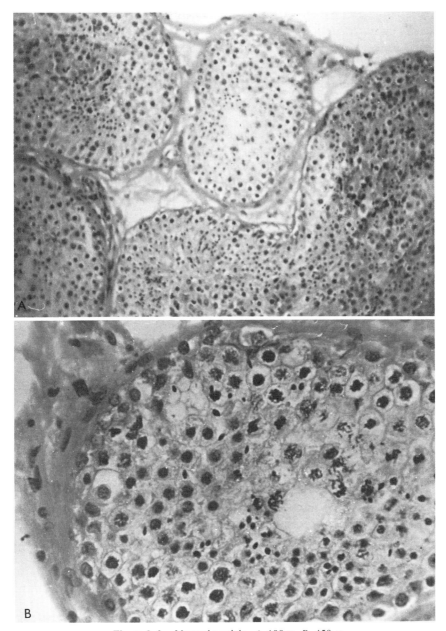

Figure 8–2.   Normal testicle. *A*. 100 ×. *B*. 450 ×

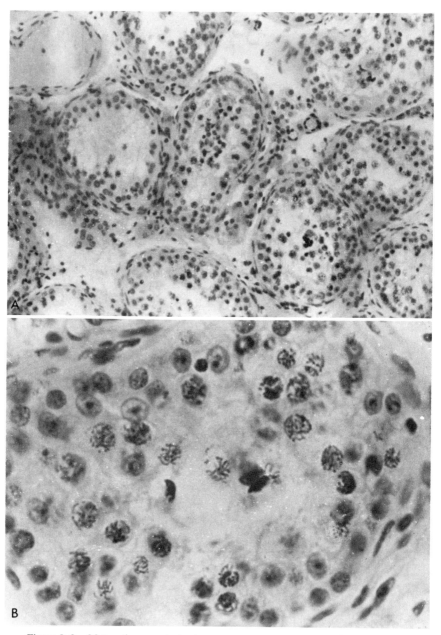

Figure 8–3. Maturation arrest at primary spermatocyte stage. *A.* 100 ×. *B.* 450 ×

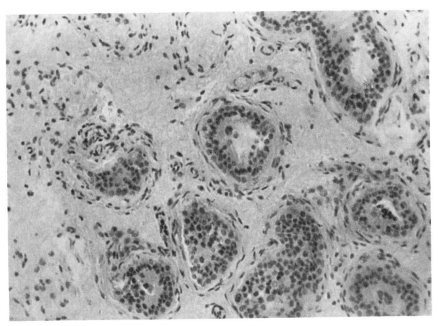

Figure 8–4. Peritubular fibrosis. 100 ×

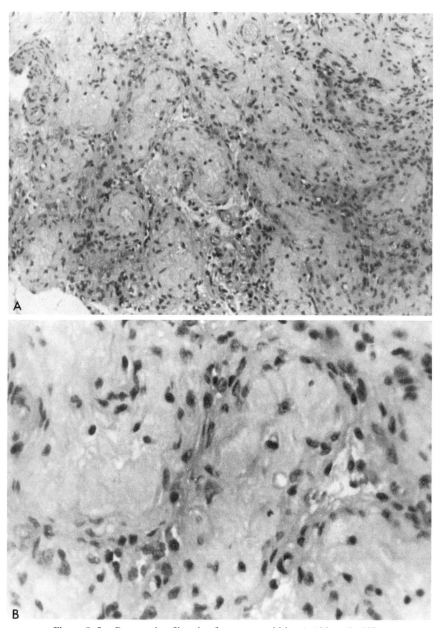

Figure 8–5. Progressive fibrosis of mumps orchitis. *A*. 100 ×. *B*. 450 ×

as mumps orchitis (Fig. 8–5) and reduced vascular supply to the testes. The testes of men with the noneunuchoid type of Klinefelter's syndrome show generalized fibrosis and hyalinization (Fig. 8–6).

Germinal Cell Aplasia and Hypoplasia. On palpation the testes of men whose azoospermia is due to germinal cell aplasia are usually normal in size and consistency. The tubules are uniform, although slightly reduced in size, and show very little peritubular fibrosis. The striking feature is the complete lack of germinal cells in the tubules, which contain only Sertoli cells (Fig. 8–7). The Leydig cells usually appear normal but occasionally show an increase in number. Serum FSH but not LH levels may be elevated. In our recent study of 1294 men with male infertility the incidence of germinal cell aplasia was 3.4 per cent, which was somewhat higher than expected.[7] It is important to make the diagnosis since no therapy is possible for this congenital condition.

In germinal cell hypoplasia there is generalized reduction in the number of germ cells of all stages (Fig. 8–8). As a result, the numbers of more mature cells are greatly reduced, and the germinal epithelium has a loose, poorly populated appearance.

Sloughing of Immature Cells. Sloughing of immature cells is a common finding in the testes of oligospermic men. In these cases the orderly pattern of spermatogenesis may be disrupted (Fig. 8–9), and immature forms, especially spermatocytes, slough into the lumina of the tubules. The seminiferous epithelium has a jumbled appearance, and many tubules contain clumps of immature cells. There may be some degree of peritubular fibrosis as well. Care must be taken not to confuse this picture with the artifacts that occur in biopsies that have received rough handling; the germinal epithelium is fragile, and the subsequent crushing and detaching of cells from the tubular walls may give the appearance of sloughing.

This picture is characteristic of varicocele as previously described in Chapter 3. Progressive sloughing will also produce the appearance of germinal cell hypoplasia due to depletion of the seminiferous tubules.[8]

OTHER CONDITIONS FOUND ON TESTICULAR BIOPSY

Hypogonadotropic Eunuchoidism. Although most eunuchoid patients appear similar in body configuration and lack of secondary sexual development, the histologic picture of biopsy specimens from these patients may vary considerably. The testicular condition most commonly found in eunuchoid men is failure of tubular and Leydig cell maturation due to lack of adequate stimulation by pituitary gonadotropins. Serum FSH, LH, and testosterone levels are low. In this group of men, initiation of testicular activity by gonadotropins, particularly androgen production, is sometimes followed by spontaneous and continued testicular activity when treatment is withdrawn.

Text continued on page 174

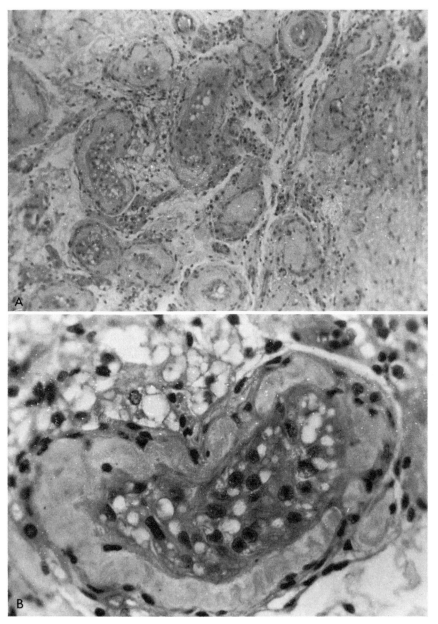

Figure 8–6. Klinefelter's syndrome. *A*. 100 ×. *B*. 450 ×

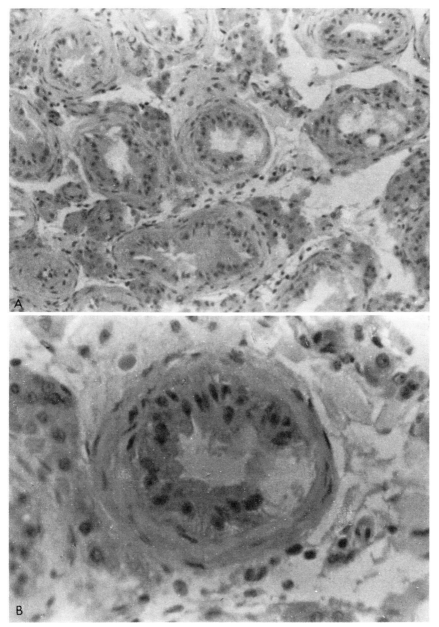

Figure 8–7. Germinal cell aplasia. *A*. 100 ×. *B*. 450 ×

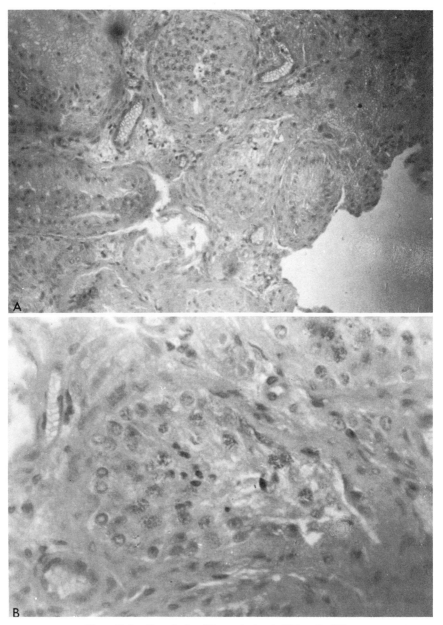

Figure 8–8.   Germinal cell hypoplasia. *A*. 100 ×. *B*. 450 ×

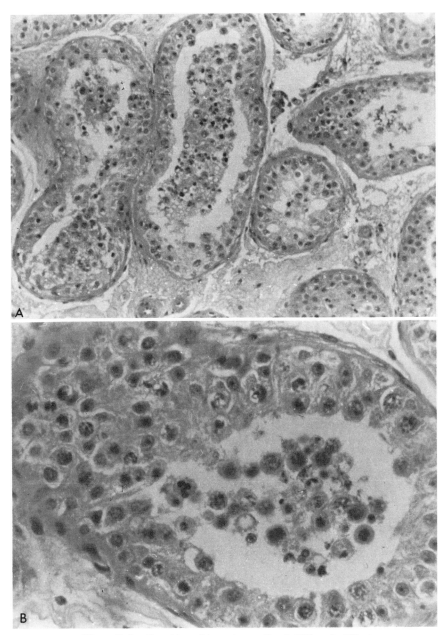

Figure 8–9. Sloughing of immature cells. *A*. 100 ×. *B*. 450 ×

Klinefelter's Syndrome (Fig. 8–6).   This syndrome is an unusual clinical entity that was first described by Klinefelter, Reifenstein, and Albright in 1942.[15] It occurred in 2.7 per cent of the series of men we reported in 1971.[7]

As originally described, it was characterized by high FSH excretion, normal 17-ketosteroid and estrogen excretion, gynecomastia in most patients, a tendency toward eunuchoidal build with increased fat distribution in the trochanteric areas, and azoospermia with hyalinization of the tubules. The Leydig cells appear normal or increased in number.

It has been demonstrated that about 75 per cent of patients with Klinefelter's syndrome have a positive chromatin pattern. A positive chromatin pattern in a phenotypic male is pathognomonic of Klinefelter's syndrome. Indeed, early recognition of the syndrome in infants or very young boys is possible by a study of the chromatin pattern before any of the classical stigmata are evident.[4] However, an individual with a negative chromatin pattern, azoospermic small testes with tubular hyalinization and normal or increased Leydig cells, and high FSH and normal 17-ketosteroid excretion with or without gynecomastia would also be classified in the same syndrome. The patient with the positive chromatin pattern may be described as having a gonadal dysplasia.

Myotonic Muscular Dystrophy.   Testicular atrophy occurs in at least 80 per cent of males who have myotonic muscular dystrophy.[6] The atrophy seems to involve the seminiferous tubules, the function of the Leydig cells being grossly normal. The testicular lesion is considered primary and not the result of anterior pituitary failure. The testicular lesion differs morphologically from that of Klinefelter's syndrome in that some spermatogenic activity is usually present. Histologic study of the testes in myotonia shows disorganization of spermatogenesis followed by a progressive decrease in spermatogenic activity, degeneration of germinal and Sertoli cells, peritubular fibrosis, and complete tubular sclerosis.

Miscellaneous Conditions.   Inadvertently, one may find evidence of lymphoma, arteritis, or inflammatory disease in testicular biopsies. Indeed, when periarteritis nodosa is suspected clinically, a biopsy of the testicular area is an excellent means of confirming the characteristic vascular lesions.

Occasional biopsies may show all elements of spermatogenesis, but there may be germinal disorganization of the orderly spermatogenic patterns.

REFERENCES

1. Amelar, R. D.: Infertility in Men: Diagnosis and Treatment. Philadelphia, F. A. Davis Co., 1966, Chapter 5.
2. Amelar, R. D., and Dubin, L.: Infertility in the male. Practice of Surgery. Vol. 2, Urology. New York, Harper and Row, 1971.
3. Amelar, R. D., and Dubin, L.: Male infertility: current diagnosis and treatment. Urology, *1*:1, 1973.

4. Briggs, D. K., Epstein, J. A., and Kupperman, H. S.: The place of chromatin sex determinations in Klinefelter's syndrome. J. Clin. Endocrinol., *16*:689, 1956.
5. Charny, C. W.: Reflections on testicular biopsy. Fertil. Steril., *14*:610, 1963.
6. Drucker, W. D., Blang, W. A., Rowland, L. P., Grumbach, N. M., and Christy, N. P.: Testes in myotonic muscular dystrophy: clinical and pathologic study, with comparison with Klinefelter's syndrome. J. Clin. Endocrinol., *23*:59, 1963.
7. Dubin, L., and Amelar, R. D.: Etiologic factors in 1294 consecutive cases of male infertility. Fertil. Steril., *22*:469, 1971.
8. Dubin, L., and Hotchkiss, R. S.: Testis biopsy in subfertile men with varicocele. Fertil. Steril., *20*:1:50, 1969.
9. Engle, E. T.: The testis biopsy in infertility. J. Urol., *57*:789, 1947.
10. Getzoff, P. L.: Testicular biopsy evaluation of the infertile male. Transactions American Urologic Association, Southeastern Section, 1956, pp. 60–70.
11. Girgis, S. M., Etriby, A., Ibrahim, A. A., and Kahil, S. A.: Testicular biopsy in azoospermia: a review of the last 10 years' experience of over 800 cases. Fertil. Steril., *20*:467, 1969.
12. Gordon, D. L., Barr, A. B., Herrigel, J. E., and Paulsen, C. A.: Testicular biopsy in men. Effect upon sperm concentration. Fertil. Steril., *16*:522, 1965.
13. Heller, C. G., and Clemont, Y.: Kinetics of the germinal epithelium in man. Rec. Progr. Hormone Res., *20*:545, 1964.
14. Heller, C. G., Nelson, W. O., Hill, I. B., Henderson, E., Maddock, W. O., Jungck, E. C., Paulsen, C. A., and Mortimore, G. E.: Improvement in spermatogenesis following depression of the human testis with testosterone. Fertil. Steril., *1*:415, 1950.
15. Klinefelter, H. F., Jr., Reifenstein, E. G., Jr., and Albright, F.: Syndrome characterized by gynecomastia, aspermatogenesis without aleydigism and increased excretion of follicle-stimulating hormone. J. Clin. Endocrinol., *2*:615, 1942.
16. Nelson, W. O.: Testicular morphology in eunuchoidal and infertile men. Fertil. Steril., *1*:477, 1950.
17. Nelson, W. O., and Heller, C. G.: Hyalinization of seminiferous tubules associated with normal or failing Leydig cell function. J. Clin. Endocrinol., *5*:13, 1945.
18. Rowley, M. J., and Heller, C. G.: The testicular biopsy: surgical procedure, fixation and staining techniques. Fertil. Steril., *17*:177, 1966.
19. Rowley, M. J., O'Keefe, K. B., and Heller, C. G.: Decreases in sperm concentration due to testicular biopsy procedures in man. J. Urol., *101*:347, 1969.

Part *III*

THERAPY OF MALE INFERTILITY

Chapter 9

MEDICAL MANAGEMENT OF MALE INFERTILITY

Patrick C. Walsh, M.D.
Richard D. Amelar, M.D.

THERAPY OF SPECIFIC ENDOCRINE DISORDERS

In the management of the infertile male, specific endocrine therapy can be utilized to induce sexual maturation and spermatogenesis in patients with gonadotropin deficiency. In patients with irreversible damage to the seminiferous tubules and Leydig cells, specific endocrine therapy is necessary for replacement of androgenic steroids. The principles underlying the management of these two major types of disorders are discussed in the first part of this chapter.

GONADOTROPIN THERAPY

For the initiation of mature spermatogenesis in mammalian species, both luteinizing hormone (LH) and follicle-stimulating hormone (FSH) are

179

necessary. Steinberger has provided an excellent review that summarizes the experimental evidence concerning the hormonal requirements necessary for the initiation of spermatogenesis.[43] He found that hormones are not required for the formation of either type A and B spermatogonia or primary spermatocytes, nor is it necessary for the progression of the meiotic prophase. However, for the maturation of late primary spermatocytes to mature spermatozoa, two hormones act sequentially: testosterone (synthesized by the Leydig cells under the regulation of LH) and FSH. Testosterone acts earliest, stimulating primary spermatocytes to divide to form secondary spermatocytes. Testosterone must be present in high local concentrations to exert this influence. This high concentration is possible because of the anatomic location of the Leydig cells just a few microns from the germinal epithelium. Finally, FSH acts to induce maturation of late spermatids to mature spermatozoa. Once spermatogenesis is initiated, it is unclear whether FSH is necessary to maintain spermatogenesis; if FSH is necessary, it may be necessary only in small amounts (see Chapter 1).

In man, gonadotropin deficiency may be caused by one of a variety of disorders involving the hypothalamic-pituitary axis. These disorders give rise to a failure of LH and FSH secretion from the pituitary. If this occurs prior to puberty, sexual maturation fails to occur, and histologically the testes demonstrate immature seminiferous tubules containing many undifferentiated germinal elements with occasional early spermatogonia and absent Leydig cells. If gonadotropin deficiency occurs after puberty—e.g., posthypophysectomy—the man will develop loss of libido and potentia, a reduction in ejaculate volume, and small, soft testes. Histologically, instead of reverting to the prepubertal state, the testes show successively maturation arrest, loss of germ cells, reduction in diameter of the tubules, and progressive thickening and hyalinization of the tunica propria.[47] In many instances, the testes become completely hyalinized, and the Leydig cells progressively decrease in number and show degenerative changes. If gonadotropin therapy is to reinitiate spermatogenesis after hypophysectomy, it must be given before the testes are completely hyalinized.

Several gonadotropin preparations have been utilized in the management of these disorders: human hypophyseal gonadotropin (HPG), human menopausal gonadotropin (HMG), human chorionic gonadotropin (HCG), human pituitary LH (HLH), and human pituitary FSH (HFSH). Because of the difficulty of obtaining a sufficient number of human pituitaries, HPG preparations are not commercially available.[38, 39] Since 1968, highly purified HLH and HFSH preparations have been available upon request for clinical investigation from the National Pituitary Agency, the National Institute of Arthritis, Metabolism and Digestive Diseases, and the National Institutes of Health in Bethesda, Maryland. However, most clinical studies have utilized HMG and HCG. HMG is commercially available as Pergonal (menotropins), supplied by Serono Laboratories in ampules containing 75 I.U. of FSH activity and 75 I.U. of LH activity. At the present time this preparation is approved for the treatment of female infertility but is considered an investigational drug in the treatment of male hypogonadism.[38, 39] HCG is commercially available as APL (chorionic gonadotropin) supplied by Ayerst Laboratories in Secules containing 5000, 10,000, and 20,000 U.S.P. units and as Follutein (chorionic gonadotropin) supplied by E. R. Squibb and Sons in vials containing 10,000 U.S.P. units.

Rosenberg has provided a recent summary of the results of gonadotropin therapy in hypogonadotropism.[38, 39] In a review of the published literature, she found that combined therapy with HCG and HMG induced complete gonadal maturation in all hypophysectomized patients and in 14 of the 17 eunuchoidal patients treated. In these studies she found that the use of HMG or HPG alone in most instances induced stimulation of the germinal epithelium to the spermatocyte stage and occasionally restored spermatogenesis. HCG therapy alone stimulated the spermatogonial phase, giving rise to spermatids and spermatocytes, stimulation of the Sertoli cells, and enlargement of the Leydig cells. In hypophysectomized or hypogonadotropic eunuchoidal patients, combined HMG–HCG therapy or HPG–HCG therapy resulted in complete gonadal maturation. However, the length of time in therapy necessary to bring about complete restoration of spermatogenesis varied from $1\frac{1}{2}$ to 12 months. After spermatogenesis was initiated, it could be maintained by HCG therapy alone.

Because Kallman's syndrome is due to an absence of GnRH, it is reasonable to assume that treatment of this disorder with GnRH may induce sexual maturation and spermatogenesis. Because synthetic GnRH has been available for only a short time, long-term results of treatment are not available. However, Mortimer and co-workers have recently reported encouraging results in the management of patients with hypogonadotropism due to diseases of the hypothalamus or pituitary.[30] In this study, 12 male patients with clinical hypogonadism due to hypothalamic or pituitary disease were treated with synthetic GnRH, 500 μg. every 8 hours for up to 1 year. Potency returned in all adult patients, and spermatogenesis was induced and maintained in the four patients who received treatment for more than 4 months. At present, GnRH is not available for routine clinical use, and because of its short half-life in the serum, it must be injected at frequent intervals. It is to be hoped that, with the development of a long-acting form of this agent, treatment with GnRH may replace the more expensive conventional use of gonadotropin replacement in patients with Kallman's syndrome.

ANDROGEN REPLACEMENT

In the treatment of hypogonadal patients with primary testicular failure, the intramuscular administration of the long-acting esters of testosterone (cypionate or enanthate) appears to be the most effective means for both the induction of sexual maturation and the maintenance of virilization. Unfortunately, testosterone is not very effective when taken by mouth because of its rapid metabolism by the liver.[33] To reduce the rapid metabolic clearance of orally administered testosterone, a variety of 17α substitutions have been utilized, for example, 17α-methyltestosterone. However, the serum half-life of 17α-methyltestosterone is only 2.7 hours,[2] and when administered in doses of 75 to 100 mg. per day this agent is associated with cholestatic jaundice.[10] In addition, there have been reports of the development of peliosis hepatis[3] or hepatic carcinoma[17] in patients receiving 17α-substituted androgens.

Consequently, the injectable forms of testosterone appear to be the safest effective agents for the induction and maintenance of virilization. An obvious disadvantage of this form of therapy is the necessity for intramuscular administration. However, when testosterone enanthate is administered intramuscularly in a dose of 200 mg., blood levels of testosterone are maintained for 2 to 4 weeks.[1] Treatment is usually initiated with bimonthly injections of 200 mg. until the desired result is achieved. At this time, the interval between doses can often be left to the discretion of the patient, since these patients are sensitive to the subtle alterations in libido and aggressive behavior that wane as the blood level of testosterone falls. Based on these subjective feelings they can usually titrate themselves appropriately.

NONSPECIFIC (EMPIRICAL) THERAPY IN PATIENTS WITHOUT ENDOCRINOPATHY

In the great majority of infertile men, a definite endocrine abnormality cannot be identified. However, it is entirely possible that in some patients there may be quantitative endocrine deficiencies, e.g., subclinical hypothalamic-pituitary disease, that cannot be detected with present laboratory tests but may be responsible for varying degrees of oligospermia or abnormal sperm maturation. On this basis, many investigators have attempted to treat men with idiopathic oligospermia in the hope of correcting subclinical endocrine deficiencies. These forms of therapy will be reviewed.

THYROID THERAPY

In this age of scientific medicine a variety of tests that can accurately define the metabolic status of a patient are readily available, and there is no place in the treatment of male infertility for the empirical use of thyroid medication in men with normal thyroid function. We have been unimpressed by the reputed efficacy of thyroid therapy, particularly Ltriiodothyronine (Cytomel), in causing improvement in a subfertile semen specimen in a euthyroid patient.

THE REBOUND PHENOMENON

The "testosterone rebound phenomenon" was first observed in patients with normal testes by Heller et al.,[14] and was used in treating patients first by Heckel[13] and later by Charny.[6] This treatment is based on inhibiting endogenous pituitary gonadotropic hormone secretion with high doses of androgens, with consequent depression of spermatogenesis to the point of azoospermia. Cessation of the androgen treatment is followed by the release of stored-up gonadotropins which promote a resurgence of spermatogenesis to higher than pretreatment levels. Our experience with this form of therapy has been disappointing because most of the patients have not rebounded but have had severe and in some cases even permanent depression of sperm counts. Patients with severe oligospermia should be warned that with this treatment sperm may not be found again in the semen for months or years once the depression takes place.[19] Few patients are willing to take such a risk. We have, therefore reserved the use of this therapy for those patients who have severe oligospermia which is refractory to all other forms of treatment and whose testicular biopsies reveal no fibrosis or sclerosis. Depo-testosterone 200 mg. weekly for 12 weeks has been used. This is usually more than enough to produce azoospermia. Spermatozoa usually return to the ejaculate within 4 to 6 months and rise to a new height in about 20 per cent of these carefully selected patients. However, even in those who are benefited, the duration of the improvement in sperm count generally lasts only a month or two, after which the sperm count drops rapidly to or below the pretreatment level. Charny[6] has recommended repeated courses of testosterone therapy if the first course does not yield a satisfactory rebound. He has reported improvement in 3 out of 21 men who were initially azoospermic. The sperm concentrations in these men rose temporarily to 47 million, 42.3 million, and 24.7 million per ml., respectively, after repeated courses of testosterone administration.

Rowley and Heller reported enthusiastically on their excellent results with the rebound phenomenon[40] and stated that the failure of others to obtain similar results was due to not following their "recipe" exactly. They stipulated that the therapy must consist of oral norethandrolone tablets (Nilevar) 10 mg. twice daily for 10 weeks and testosterone enanthate (Delatestryl) 200 mg. intramuscularly on the first day of therapy and again at the third and sixth weeks of therapy. Suppression to azoospermic levels must occur, following which there is often a temporary rebound to normal levels.

Unfortunately, Nilevar was withdrawn from the market shortly before the paper was published, and other clinicians have not had the opportunity to test this therapeutic regimen.

LOW DOSAGE ANDROGEN THERAPY

Exogenous androgen administration can suppress endogenous gonadotropin release and thus suppress sperm production. It has been postulated that small doses of orally administered androgens can at times be a useful form of therapy in patients without demonstrable endocrinopathy who have the unusual combination of poor sperm motility associated with good sperm count and normal sperm morphology.[23] MacLeod has reasoned that poor sperm motility in the ejaculate may be due to a failure of the epididymis in particular and of the ductal epithelium as a whole to supply the support which appears to be necessary not only for full maturation of the spermatozoa subsequent to their release from the germinal epithelium but also during their long passage through the duct system. Since the epithelium of the male duct system depends upon the hormone activity of the Leydig cells for their secretory activity, it is possible that a partial or total failure of Leydig cell activity or a failure of the epithelium to utilize the available hormone properly may occur. According to MacLeod's reasoning, either of these failures would lead to inadequate support of the spermatozoa in the duct system and a consequent failure of the spermatozoa to show good motility in the ejaculate. The epithelial failure need not and probably does not induce defects in head shape in the spermatozoa. In the past, MacLeod suggested treatment with exogenous testosterone, such as 10 to 25 mg. of methyl testosterone once or twice daily in patients who show a significant decrease in sperm motility. After methyl testosterone was shown to be hepatotoxic, another oral androgen, fluoxymesterone (Halotestin), was recommended in doses of 10 mg. twice daily. In the series recently reported by Brown,[5] 30 of 58 infertile men (52 per cent) who had poor sperm motility combined with good sperm count and morphology showed improvement after a course of fluoxymesterone 10 mg. twice a day for 6 weeks, and 12 (20 per cent) of the 58 maintained their improved motility for at least 3 months after cessation of therapy.

It is thought that these doses will not inhibit pituitary gonadotropin, thus maintaining the sperm count, but it has been our experience that the sperm count should be watched carefully while the patient is receiving exogenous androgen because some patients have developed spermatogenic depression even at this dosage level. We have employed even smaller doses, namely 5 and 10 mg. of Halotestin once on alternate days.

HUMAN CHORIONIC GONADOTROPIN (HCG) THERAPY

Another, perhaps more physiologic, approach to therapy for poor sperm motility was advocated by Misurale et al.,[29] who used injections of human chorionic gonadotropin 2500 I.U. intramuscularly every 5 days for 75 days to 90 days. They reported an improvement in sperm motility in 16 of 17 patients treated, and eight pregnancies occurred in six of the wives of the patients treated.

The theory that Leydig cell failure leads to poor sperm motility has been supported by MacLeod.[24] Hypophysectomy is now being performed in males in the reproductive age group for the treatment of diabetic retinopathy, and MacLeod has had the opportunity of studying semen quality prior to hypophysectomy and at intervals thereafter during the process of involution of the reproductive system which inevitably follows if the hypophysectomy is complete. In the patients he studied, the semen quality was excellent prior to the operation. In the first specimens, which were seen 3 weeks postoperatively, the sperm counts remained relatively high (since there had been no intervening emissions these cells were present in the duct system prior to operation), but the ejaculate volumes were markedly reduced. The most impressive postoperative reaction, however, was the complete absence of sperm motility. Within 5 weeks after the operation the ejaculate had disappeared, even though normal erection and orgasm were maintained.

If, as seems certain, LH activity in the blood stream (which is necessary for Leydig cell maintenance) disappeared rapidly after hypophysectomy, the appropriate hormone support for the ductal epithelium would also have been withdrawn. MacLeod has demonstrated that the administration of human pituitary gonadotropin and chorionic gonadotropin restored all these deficiencies in these hypophysectomized males, including sperm motility.

Although the commercially obtainable preparations of human chorionic gonadotropin have primarily LH activity, they may also have a small amount of FSH activity,[3, 4] and this may be responsible for the success noted in the treatment of idiopathic oligospermia with HCG injections.[9, 12, 29]

We have employed human chorionic gonadotropin injection therapy empirically in patients with idiopathic oligospermia, and after varicocelectomy in those patients who had preoperative sperm concentrations below 10 million per ml.[7] All of these patients had poor sperm motility and morphology as well as low sperm counts. We use doses of 4000 units intramuscularly twice a week for 10 weeks. Semen improvement can be expected starting about 3 months after the completion of the injection series; in some of the patients this will be preceded by an initial decrease in semen quality. A frequently noted side effect of HCG therapy is an increase in libido with an improvement in the quality of sexual performance reported by the patient. Indeed, this effect on sexual performance is remarkably constant and may at times justify the use of HCG therapy in patients with impotence, even though they may not have any problems with semen quality.

An uncommon side effect is transient nipple tenderness and gynecomastia, which are noted in less than 5 per cent of patients toward the end of the course of therapy; it disappears when therapy is stopped. There will be a transient rise in plasma testosterone levels during therapy with HCG in those patients with intact Leydig cell function.

HUMAN MENOPAUSAL GONADOTROPIN (HMG) THERAPY

The use of human menopausal gonadotropin (Pergonal), which has primarily FSH-like activity, either with or without combined therapy with human chorionic gonadotropin (HCG), has had little clinical trial in the United States because it is not generally available and is considerably expensive; in addition, because the Food and Drug Administration has not formally approved its use in men, it is in the category of an experimental drug, and special consent is required for its clinical use. Lytton and Mroueh reported poor results when HMG therapy was used empirically for idiopathic oligospermia.[21]

Abroad, a very low success rate has been reported by Lunenfeld et al. — only one pregnancy resulted after 80 to 120 days of therapy in their 51 oligospermic patients.[20] Similarly, Polishuk et al. were disappointed with the poor results obtained from combined HMG and HCG therapy.[37]

In an attempt to improve these poor results, which may be due to poor selection of patients for therapy, Schwarzstein[42] in Argentina performed testicular biopsies on 12 men with idiopathic oligospermia and then treated them with injections of HMG and HCG three times a week for up to 270 days. He found that in six patients who had only minimal alterations in spermatogenesis at the spermatid level the results of therapy were better than in the six patients with more severe alterations in spermatogenesis; thus the more normal testicular biopsy, the better the result. However, the small size of the series did not allow determination of optimal dose levels.

CORTISONE THERAPY

For many years, numerous investigators have been attracted by the study of the action of adrenal corticoids on spermatogenesis in man. Various results have been obtained using different types and doses of hormones and varying the length of time administration. Some patients with different degrees of idiopathic oligospermia showed a transitory improvement in sperm count,[16, 25, 28, 46] while other patients with similar abnormalities showed no changes or even a decrease in sperm count.[16, 22, 25, 28]

In a study employing large and small doses of prednisolone, a synthetic corticosteroid, Mancini et al.[26] found that a severe depression in spermatogenesis occurred in all patients receiving 30 mg. of the hormone daily for 4 weeks, with recovery to pretreatment levels only 6 months after the treatment. Patients receiving doses of 10 mg. daily did not show any substantial changes in sperm count.

Stewart[24] has suggested that cortisone acetate in a low dose range of 2.5 to 5 mg. four times daily for up to 12 months may be the "nonspecific treatment of choice" in most cases of idiopathic oligospermia. However, our own experience indicates that the indiscriminate use of cortisone therapy in males with idiopathic oligospermia is unwise; cortisone should be reserved for suppression of the adrenal cortex in patients with oligospermia secondary to the adrenogenital syndrome.

CLOMIPHENE THERAPY

Gonadotropin stimulation of the subfertile testes can be obtained by administering exogenous gonadotropins as well as by stimulating endogenous gonadotropin release. The latter phenomenon can be produced by administering clomiphene citrate (Clomid) to oligospermic males with normal or low control gonadotropin levels. The increase in gonadotropin secretion that results is produced by blocking the negative feedback of testicular steroids on the pituitary, with consequent rise in LH and FSH levels.

The increase in gonadotropins involves both FSH and LH moieties and is associated in the male with increased levels of urinary 17-keto-steroids and estrogen, whereas 17-hydroxysteroid levels remain unchanged. These observations, plus the fact that a rise in urinary 17-ketosteroids does not occur in women treated with clomiphene citrate, indicate that these urinary steroid responses are caused by Leydig cell stimulation by LH and not by adrenocortical stimulation. The augmentation of FSH release with clomiphene citrate produced slight to marked increases in sperm counts in 10 of 13 oligospermic patients studied by Mellinger and Thompson.[27] Sperm response was not maintained, however, with continued therapy; sperm motility was not improved; and there were no conceptions during or after the treatment. Mroueh, Lytton, and Kase[31] found improvement in only 1 of 15 oligospermic patients treated with 50 mg. of clomiphene citrate per day for 6 weeks, but semen counts in these patients were done only 2 to 4 weeks after completion of therapy.

Palti[35] suggested that the dose of clomiphene should be 50 mg. daily for 60 days; he reported five pregnancies occurring in the wives of 69 patients treated. Paulson and Wacksman[36] recently reported favorable results using a dose of 25 mg. clomiphene citrate per day for a 25-day cycle with 5-day rest periods, maintaining therapy for up to 9 months. They reported 35 hypofertile males who had assays of serum FSH, LH, and testosterone. No relationship could be established between FSH levels and sperm counts in this group of patients, but total sperm counts were improved in 31 men while they were on therapy, and eight pregnancies occurred among the patients' wives. Paulson and Wacksman also reported on the treatment of 10 oligospermic males who had testicular biopsies prior to therapy. In three of these patients the biopsies were completely normal, and these were the only patients who showed an elevation of total sperm count with clomiphene treatment. These patients also showed no significant rise in FSH levels while receiving the therapy. In other patients, biopsies showed some abnormality (such as basement membrane thickening with tubular hyalinization, hypospermatogenesis, maturation arrest, or sparse tubules with loose stroma, among other findings), the sperm count did not increase during treatment, but the FSH levels did show a marked increase during clomiphene therapy. There was only one pregnancy among the patients' wives in this group, and that patient refused further study after his wife became pregnant.

Some patients who receive therapy with clomiphene citrate show an early increase in sperm count followed by a decline during continuation of the therapy.

In general, the semen responses of oligospermic men to clomiphene citrate have been very unpredictable and inadequately studied. Whether the variation in reported results is caused by the use of different doses, different duration of therapeutic courses, or inadequate follow-up of seminal response is still in question.

Epstein, in a still unpublished study,[8] has used interrupted Clomid therapy, 100 mg. three times a week, in an attempt to avoid overstimulation of the Leydig cells with resultant spermatogenic depression, but there are insufficient data at present to evaluate this treatment schedule.

As a practical point for the physician, the use of clomiphene citrate therapy in the oligospermic male must at present be considered experimental, and an informed consent must be obtained from the patient. By current regulation of the U.S. Food and Drug Administration, clomiphene should be used solely for the induction of ovulation in women with ovulatory failure who desire pregnancy. The use of clomiphene citrate in males has not yet been approved by the F.D.A.

It is possible that clomiphene citrate may have a place in the treatment of otherwise unexplained oligospermia in patients with low or low–normal FSH levels, low–normal urinary 17-ketosteroid excretion levels, and low–normal testosterone levels. The suggested dose of clomiphene is 50 to 100 mg. (one or two 50 mg. tablets) three times weekly. While taking the medication the patient should have monthly follow-up semen analyses (at the time of the wife's menses, so as not to interfere with attempts at conception) and monthly assays of FSH and testosterone levels. The therapy should be stopped after 6 months if there has been no improvement in semen quality, if a marked rise in FSH or testosterone occurs, or if there is a worsening of the semen quality after early improvement. Therapy should also be stopped if the patient develops visual symptoms such as blurring of vision or scintillating scotomata.

ARGININE THERAPY

As discussed in Chapter 4, several amino acids have been used, with varying degrees of reported success, to treat cases of oligospermia and asthenospermia. Of the amino acids utilized for this purpose, arginine has received the most attention, and there have been several reports of encouraging results.[4, 11, 15, 41, 45] However, these reports do not hold up under critical analysis.[18]

Our own experience coincides with that of Mroueh,[32] who found no improvement in semen quality regardless of pathology in patients given 2 grams of arginine hydrochloride daily for 10 weeks, and with that of Jungling and Bunge,[18] who reported that the daily oral administration of 4 grams of arginine was of no benefit in patients with spermatogenic maturation arrest. We do not believe that arginine therapy is an effective approach to the improvement of poor semen quality.

REFERENCES

1. Aakvaag, A., and Vogt, J. H.: Plasma testosterone values in different forms of testosterone treatment. Acta. Endocrinol., 60:537, 1969.
2. Alkalay, D., Khemani, L., Wagner, W. E., Jr. et al.: Sublingual and oral administration of methyltestosterone: a comparison of drug bioavailability. J. Clin. Pharmacol., 13:142, 1973.
3. Bagheri, S. A., and Boyer, J. L.: Peliosis hepatis associated with androgenic-anabolic steroid therapy: a severe form of hepatic injury. Ann. Intern. Med., 81:610, 1974.
4. Bernard, I.: Treatment of oligoasthenospermia with arginine. In Western, B., and Wiquist, N. (eds.): Proceedings of the Fifth World Congress on Fertility and Sterility. Stockholm, June 16–22, 1966. Amsterdam, Excerpta Medica Foundation, 1967, p. 898.
5. Brown, J. S.: The effect of orally administered androgens on sperm motility. Fertil. Steril., 26:305, 1975.
6. Charny, C. W.: The use of androgens for human spermatogenesis. Fertil. Steril., 10:557, 1959.
7. Dubin, L., and Amelar, R. D.: Varicocelectomy as therapy in male infertility: a study of 504 cases. Fertil. Steril., 26:217, 1975.
8. Epstein, J. E.: Personal communication, 1976.
9. Futterweit, W., and Sobrero, A. J.: Treatment of normogonadotrophic oligospermia with large doses of chorionic gonadotrophin. Fertil. Steril., 19:971, 1968.
10. Gardner, F. H., and Pringle, J. C.: Androgens and erythropoiesis. I. Preliminary clinical observations. Arch. Intern. Med., 107:846, 1961.
11. Giarola, A., and Agostine, G.: Amino acids in the treatment of male sterility. In Westen, B., and Wiqvist, N. (eds.): Proceedings of the Fifth World Congress on Fertility and Sterility, Stockholm, June 16–22, 1966. Amsterdam, Excerpta Medica Foundation, 1967, p. 892.
12. Glass, S. J., and Holland, H. M.: Treatment of oligospermia with large doses of human chorionic gonadotropin. Fertil. Steril., 14:500, 1963.
13. Heckel, N. J., Rosso, W. A., and Kestel, L.: Spermatogenic rebound phenomenon after testosterone therapy. J. Clin. Endocrinol., 2:235, 1951.
14. Heller, C. G., Nelson, W. O., Hill, I. B., et al.: Improvement in spermatogenesis following depression of the human testes with testosterone. Fertil. Steril., 1:415, 1950.
15. Ishigami, J.: Non-endocrine drugs in the treatment of male infertility. Excerpta Medica Int. Congr. Ser. 109. Amsterdam, Excerpta Medica, 1966.
16. Jefferies, W. M., Weir, W. C., Weir, D. R., and Prouty, R. L.: The use of cortisone and related steroids in infertility. Fertil. Steril., 9:145, 1958.
17. Johnson, F. L., Feagler, J. R., Lerner, K. G., et al.: Association of androgenic-anabolic steroid therapy with development of hepatocellular carcinoma. Lancet, 2:1213, 1972.

18. Jungling, M. L., and Bunge, R. G.: The treatment of spermatogenic arrest with arginine. Fertil. Steril., *27*:282, 1976.
19. Lamesdorf, H., Compere, D., and Begley, G.: Testosterone rebound in the treatment of male infertility. Fertil. Steril., *26*:469, 1975.
20. Lunenfeld, B., Mor, A., and Mani, M.: Treatment of male infertility. 1. Human gonadotropins (Pergonal). Fertil. Steril., *18*:581, 1967.
21. Lytton, B., and Mroueh, A.: Treatment of oligospermia with urinary human menopausal gonadotropin: a preliminary report. Fertil. Steril., *17*:696, 1966.
22. McDonald, J. H., and Heckel, N. J.: The effect of cortisone on the spermatogenic function of the human testes. J. Urol., *75*:527, 1956.
23. MacLeod, J.: The semen examination. Clin. Obstet. Gynecol., *8*:115, 1965.
24. MacLeod, J., Pazianos, A., and Ray, B.: Restoration of human spermatogenesis by menopausal gonadotropins. Lancet, *1*:1196, 1964.
25. Maddock, W. O., Chase, J. D., and Nelson, W.: The effects of large doses of cortisone on testicular morphology and urinary gonadotrophin, estrogen and 17-ketosteroid excretion. J. Lab. Clin. Med., *1*:608, 1953.
26. Mancini, R. E., Lavieri, J. C., Muller, F., Andrada, J. A., and Saraceni, D. J.: Effect of prednisolone on normal and pathologic human spermatogenesis. Fertil. Steril., *17*:500, 1966.
27. Mellinger, R. C., and Thompson, R. J.: The effect of clomiphene citrate in male infertility. Fertil. Steril., *17*:94, 1966.
28. Michelson, L., Roland, S., and Koets, P.: The effects of cortisone on the infertile male. Fertil. Steril., *6*:493, 1955.
29. Misurale, F., Cagnazzo, C., and Storace, A.: Asthenospermia and its treatment with HCG. Fertil. Steril., *20*:650, 1969.
30. Mortimer, C. H., McNeilly, A. S., Fisher, R. A., Murray, M. A. F. and Besser, G. M.: Gonadotropin-releasing hormone therapy in hypogonadal males with hypothalamic or pituitary dysfunction. Brit. Med. J., *4*:617, 1974.
31. Mroueh, A., Lytton, B., and Kase, N.: Effect of clomiphene citrate on oligospermia. Amer. J. Obstet. Gynecol., *98*:1033, 1967.
32. Mroueh, A.: Effect of arginine on oligospermia. Fertil. Steril., *21*:217, 1970.
33. Murad, F., and Gilman, A. G.: Androgens and anabolic steroids. *In* Goodman, L. S., and Gillman, A. (eds.): The Pharmacological Basis of Therapeutics, 5th ed. New York, Macmillan, 1975, pp. 1451–1471.
34. Northcutt, R. C., and Albert, A.: Follicle-stimulating activity of human chorionic gonadotropin: further evidence for non-identity with follicle-stimulating hormone. J. Clin. Endocrinol. Metab., *31*:91, 1970.
35. Palti, Z.: Clomiphene therapy in defective spermatogenesis. Fertil. Steril., *21*:838, 1970.
36. Paulson, D. F., and Wacksman, J.: Clomiphene citrate in the management of male infertility. J. Urol., *115*:73, 1976.
37. Polishuk, W. Z., Palti, Z., and Laufer, A.: Treatment of defective spermatogenesis with human gonadotropins. Fertil. Steril., *18*:127, 1967.
38. Rosemberg, E.: Medical treatment of male infertility. Andrologia (Suppl.), *1*:95, 1976.
39. Rosemberg, E.: Gonadotropin therapy of male infertility, *In* Hafez, E.S.E. (ed.): Human Semen and Fertility Regulation in Men. St. Louis, C. V. Mosby Co., 1976, pp. 464–475.
40. Rowley, M. J., and Heller, C. G.: The testosterone rebound phenomenon in the treatment of male infertility. Fertil. Steril., *23*:498, 1972.
41. Schacter, A., Goldman, J. A., and Zuckerman, Z.: Treatment of oligospermia with the amino acid arginine. J. Urol., *110*:311, 1973.
42. Schwarzstein, L.: Human menopausal gonadotropins in the treatment of patients with oligospermia. Fertil. Steril., *25*:813, 1974.
43. Steinberger, E.: Hormonal control of spermatogenesis. Physiol. Rev., *51*:1, 1971.
44. Stewart, B. H.: Infertility in the male: Method of Bruce H. Stewart, M. D. *In* Conn, H. F. (ed.): Current Therapy. Philadelphia, W. B. Saunders Co., 1971.
45. Tanimura, J.: Studies on arginine in human semen. Part III. The influences of several drugs on male infertility. Bull. Osaka Med. Schl., *13*:90, 1967.
46. Trabucco, A.: Ensayo de cortisona en el tratamiento de las oligozoospermias de tercer grade. Obstet. Ginec. Lat. Amer., *10*:511, 1952.
47. Wong, T. W., Straus, F. H., and Warner, N. E.: Testicular biopsy in the study of male infertility. III. Pretesticular causes of infertility. Arch. Path., *98*:1, 1974.

Chapter 10

SPECIAL PROBLEMS IN MANAGEMENT

Richard D. Amelar, M.D.
Lawrence Dubin, M.D.

If the couple is still barren after diligent medical or surgical therapy for male infertility and if no untreated female factors exist, a consideration of other techniques that may bring about a pregnancy is appropriate. This chapter is concerned with special problems contributing to infertility and methods of effectively dealing with such problems.

SEMEN VOLUME

The largest part of the seminal plasma is composed of the secretions of the seminal vesicles and prostate, the volume and content of which are under androgenic control. These secretions serve not only as a vehicle for the sperm but also as a source of nutrition and as a buffering agent protecting the sperm from the acid vaginal secretions. The spermatozoa themselves actually occupy about 0.1 per cent of the total semen volume.

In our urologic practice which has a high proportion of patient's with fertility problems, a study was made of 1294 male patients with proved subfertility.[18] A total of 11.8 per cent of these patients exhibited subfertility associated with either too low or too high a volume of semen (Table 10–1).

Table 10–1   SEMEN VOLUME IN 1294 SUBFERTILE MALES

SEMEN VOLUME	NUMBER OF CASES	PER CENT
High (>4.5 ml.)	133	10
Low (<1 ml.)	24	1.8

LOW SEMEN VOLUME

Semen with low volume (less than 1 ml.) but otherwise normal quality can lead to infertility due to failure of the seminal fluid to make contact with the cervical os and mucus.[49] Homologous insemination (AIH) with a low volume of seminal fluid can lead to pregnancy.

HIGH SEMEN VOLUME

Ten per cent of the patients had poor semen quality associated with high seminal volume (over 4.5 ml.), which may serve to dilute the sperm concentration and depress sperm motility.

THE SPLIT EJACULATE

If a semen specimen is collected in two or more containers during ejaculation, it will be found that there are significant differences between the various portions with regard to viscosity, sperm concentration, motility, and occasionally morphology compared with the total ejaculate. These differences may be profound.[3] In humans the different portions of the semen usually follow one another in a definite sequence. During ejaculation the three main glandular systems that contribute to the ejaculate discharge successively. Thus, ejaculation begins with the scant secretion of Cowper's (bulbourethral) glands, followed immediately by that from the prostate gland which contains the main bulk of the acid phosphatases. Then are added the products of the testes, epididymides, and vasa deferentia which have accumulated within the ampullary portion of the vas; this portion, therefore, contains the highest concentration of spermatozoa. The last portion of the semen contains the highest concentration of fructose, a substance specific to the seminal vesicles. The products of these three systems become more or less mixed during ejaculation.

Eliason and Lindholmer,[20] using an ingenious technique for collecting ejaculates in six fractions, also showed that spermatozoa were more highly concentrated, and had better motility and vitality in the earlier parts of split ejaculates than in later parts. Lindholmer[42] attributes the depressed sperm motility and vitality noted in the later portion of fractionated ejaculates to a suppressive factor or factors in the seminal vesicular fluid which have a deleterious effect on human sperm survival. Pedron et al.[54] found that human spermatozoa preferred glucose to fructose as a glycolytic metabolic substrate, and in the microenvironment of the female reproductive tract where fertilization takes place, glucose, not fructose, is the main carbohydrate present. It has also been postulated that a metabolic regulator released at the time of ejaculation in some manner uncouples oxidative phosphorylation, decreasing in turn the respiratory inhibition of glycolysis.[41] Pedron et al.[54] studied the differences in glycolytic metabolism of spermatozoa from normal and asthenospermic men (i.e., men in whom the sperm motility was poor but sperm count and morphology were normal). The better motility of sperm in the first fraction of the split ejaculate might be explained by a lower concentration of the metabolic uncoupling agent in the first fraction compared with the second.

COLLECTION OF SPLIT EJACULATE

To collect the split ejaculatory specimen, the patient should be given two wide-mouthed, 3 oz. ointment jars which are numbered and secured with tape to facilitate the collection. He is told to collect the first few spurts of the ejaculate in bottle number 1 and the remainder in bottle number 2. Ideally, the first third of the specimen should be put in the first bottle and the latter two-thirds in the second bottle.[7]

In a study of over 500 ejaculates of male patients attending the infertility clinic of the Margaret Sanger Research Bureau, it was found that when the ejaculate was split in this manner, the sperm count in 89 per cent was significantly higher in the first portion than in the second or in the ejaculate as a whole; in 5 per cent it was about equally distributed in both portions of the ejaculate; and in 6 per cent it was significantly higher in the second portion than in the whole ejaculate. The viscosity of the sample, sperm motility, and occasionally sperm morphology were also found to be much more favorable in the first portion than in the second.[3] Harvey,[31] in a study of partitioned ejaculates of 243 men, also found that 90 per cent had better semen quality in the first portion of the ejaculate; in six men the density and motility of the sperm were better in the second fraction.

REVERSAL OF EJACULATORY PATTERN

In 6 per cent of relatively infertile men the usual ejaculatory pattern is reversed. We refer to animal studies for elucidation of this phenomenon. In a study of stallions of proved high fertility, Mann and his co-workers[45] found that the last part of the sample, collected as a "penis drip" as the stallion dismounts after completing a service, consistently contained a much lower number of sperm per milliliter than did the earlier portion of the ejaculate. However, in a study of subfertile stallions, they found a reversal of the usual pattern of ejaculation—that is, the sperm-rich fraction was voided toward the end instead of at the beginning of ejaculation.[46] Mann attributes the alterations in ejaculatory pattern to a disturbance in the nervous mechanism that controls the normal ejaculatory sequence. Until we have more conclusive evidence from clinical studies in humans, we can only speculate that a similar defect in coordination is responsible for this phenomenon in a small percentage of infertile men.

Knowledge gained from studies on the partitioned ejaculate has bene-fitted many subfertile couples using artificial insemination (A.I.H.) of the husbands' oligospermic semen. Use of only the first portion of the split ejaculate was found to be effective in achieving pregnancies in couples in whom repeated attempts at insemination with the whole ejaculate had been unsuccessful.[3, 12, 22, 38, 76]

When the second portion of the ejaculate was demonstrated to be sig-nificantly better, it was used in inseminations to produce pregnancies.[4]

WITHDRAWAL COITAL TECHNIQUE

We have had the opportunity to evaluate in detail, using split ejacula-tion studies, over 100 subfertile men with high semen volume and good quality in the first portion of the split ejaculate with regard to sperm con-centration, motility, and morphology. However, for many of these men and their wives, artificial insemination was not always possible. Either the wife ovulated on a Saturday or Sunday when the doctor may not have been available, or the husband was not always able to produce a masturbated specimen on demand, or the couple did not wish to have insemination per-formed by a physician. There may be religious proscriptions against in-semination, as in the case of devout Catholics and orthodox Jews.

For these couples, using the phenomenon of the better first portion of the split ejaculate to therapeutic advantage, we recommended a method of sexual relations in which the husband withdraws his penis from the vagina after the coital intravaginal deposit of the first portion of the ejaculate.[8] This withdrawal coital technique should be used only around the fertile time of the wife's cycle. Furthermore, since it has been demonstrated that sperm retain their fertilizing capacity for about 2 days after ejaculation within the female reproductive tract,[30] we also recommend that the couple have sexual relations every other day rather than daily at the fertile time of the female cycle. Couples who have a poor rating on postcoital (Sims-Huener) tests when using the usual method of coitus, have demonstrated improved ratings when this method of withdrawal coitus is employed.

Table 10-2 presents a detailed analysis of the whole and partitioned ejaculates of 33 men who consulted us during the years 1970 to 1973 because of involuntarily barren marriages of many years' duration. The wives of these men became pregnant within 1 to 6 months after they began using this coital technique. In each case, the first portion of the split ejaculate was superior in quality to the specimen as a whole. Each husband submitted two whole ejaculate and two split ejaculate specimens. Data in Table 10-2 represent averages of the analysis.

It will be noted that in each case the whole ejaculate specimen would be rated subfertile,[7] indicating either low sperm density, poor motility, poor morphology, or any combination of these. Also, the first portion of the split ejaculate was superior to the specimen as a whole with regard to fertilizing potential. With the exception of Case 22, in which the wife had one tube and ovary removed prior to marriage, no obvious female factors preventing pregnancy were discovered in these wives after careful evaluation by their gynecologists. It is apparent from these *selected* cases that fractionating the ejaculate is a method of obtaining better sperm concentration in oligospermic patients. Not only were greater numbers of sperm present in the first fraction, but the motility of the sperm was significantly better in the first portion than in the second portion or the whole specimen. In each of these cases, the sperm morphology was also better in the first portion of the split ejaculate than in the whole specimen. It is emphasized that these were 33 *selected* cases; a previous study in 1965 on 86 unselected patients[3] demonstrated that the first portion of the split ejaculate had a better sperm concentration in 88.4 per cent of cases, better motility in 56 per cent, and better morphology in 20 per cent.

Our findings lend support to the theory that there is a suppressive factor or factors in the seminal vesicular fluid that causes a depression of sperm motility, which is especially obvious in men with high semen volumes. It can be argued by skeptics that (1) none of the husbands in the 33 cases was sterile; (2) in each case pregnancy was possible with ordinary coitus; and (3) the documented pregnancy could not be ascribed with assurance to the use of the technique of withdrawal after coital deposition of the first part of the ejaculate (Table 10-2). We acknowledge this possibility for any given case, but at the same time we believe that most of these couples have achieved earlier pregnancies as a result of our management. These couples sought medical help because they had barren marriages of many years' duration, and they were desperate in their desire to have children.

HIGH SEMINAL VISCOSITY

The physician is occasionally confronted with an infertile male patient in whom the problem seems to be an exceptionally high viscosity of the

Table 10–2   SEMEN ANALYSIS IN CASES OF PREGNANCY ACHIEVED WITH WITHDRAWAL COITAL TECHNIQUE (1970–1973)

Case No.	Date	WHOLE EJACULATE SPECIMEN						1ST PORTION OF SPLIT EJACULATE						2ND PORTION OF SPLIT EJACULATE						Years Trying	Months for Pregnancy
		Volume (ml) Mean	Sperm Count Millions/ml	Viscosity	Motility %	Grade	Morphology % Normal	Volume (ml) Mean	Sperm Count Millions/ml	Viscosity	Motility %	Grade	Morphology % Normal	Volume (ml) Mean	Sperm Count Millions/ml	Viscosity	Motility %	Grade	Morphology % Normal		
1	3–70	5.2	96	N	65	3	33	2.0	179	N	90	3	74	2.5	34	N	50	2	34	4	1
2	5–70	4.3	104	N	40	2+	32	1.5	168	N	60	3	58	2.8	38	N	10	1	12	5	4
3	7–70	7.3	27	1+	50	2	58	2.9	108	N	60	3	64	4.4	15	1+	20	2	49	3	3
4	7–70	5.3	45	N	55	2	65	1.0	152	N	75	2+	69	2.5	<1	N	<10	2	—	2½	2
5	8–70	6.9	19	N	50	2+	54	1.8	102	N	65	2+	72	3.3	11	N	40	2	51	2	4
6	9–70	5.2	81	N	15	2	56	1.5	151	N	60	2+	60	2.8	39	N	10	1	32	2	4
7	12–70	8.0	53	N	40	2	78	3.5	84	N	70	3	79	2.9	6	N	rare	—	46	2	1
8	1–71	6.2	22	N	60	2+	52	1.5	162	N	85	3	82	4.5	15	N	25	2	56	4	3
9	3–71	6.1	99	N	30	2	76	3.1	159	N	90	3	82	2.0	34	N	20	1	40	3	2
10	4–71	6.2	23	N	40	2	50	2.0	57	N	60	2+	66	4.1	8	N	20	2	55	6	6
11	5–71	7.1	44	N	30	2	67	2.2	90	N	55	2	75	3.4	26	N	20	1	58	2	4
12	7–71	4.5	33	N	40	2	54	1.0	88	N	50	2	76	3.2	17	N	15	2	42	2½	5

13	9-71	4.5	43	N	30	2	60	1.0	112	N	60	3	56	2.6	10	N	25	2	28	3	2
14	10-71	5.0	40	N	50	2	43	2.0	80	N	75	3	64	3.0	7	N	20	2	56	3	4
15	11-71	3.5	77	3+	40	2	61	1.0	154	1+	60	3	79	2.8	56	4+	15	1	28	4½	6
16	12-71	6.5	31	2+	30	2	72	1.1	63	N	70	3	82	5.0	3	2+	10	1	—	5	4
17	1-72	7.1	31	N	40	2	85	1.3	143	N	95	2+	88	3.5	12	N	25	2	54	4	3
18	2-72	5.4	13	N	30	2	46	1.4	56	N	70	3+	61	3.5	6	N	40	2	38	4	2
19	4-72	6.0	35	N	30	2+	66	1.3	117	N	60	3	83	5.0	14	N	10	1	48	3	3
20	4-72	5.0	61	N	50	2+	72	1.9	115	N	60	2+	73	3.0	21	N	10	1	16	2	3
21	5-72	4.2	98	N	30	2	91	1.0	150	N	60	3	88	2.4	36	N	10	1	60	1½	3
22	5-72	10.0	74	N	30	2	83	4.5	137	N	70	2+	95	6.0	22	N	15	2	85	3	2
23	6-72	7.4	106	N	30	2	54	2.0	193	N	60	3+	61	4.8	16	N	10	1	51	4	4
24	9-72	5.1	38	N	40	2	58	2.2	78	N	60	2	64	2.8	15	N	10	1	45	3	4
25	10-72	5.8	42	N	40	3	62	2.1	63	N	60	3	68	3.1	19	N	30	2	43	2	
26	1-73	5.0	35	N	30	2	60	1.5	108	N	50	2	63	3.0	13	N	15	2	40	3	4
27	2-73	5.8	81	N	40	2+	52	1.6	140	N	60	3	61	3.0	19	N	30	2	54	2	4
28	2-73	6.2	12	N	40	2+	51	2.0	47	N	50	2+	57	3.8	2	N	20	2	44	5	6
29	4-73	5.7	26	N	40	2	47	3.0	61	N	50	3	59	3.4	18	1±	10	2	39	4	5
30	5-73	5.6	26	N	40	2+	62	2.1	67	N	60	3	65	3.0	9	N	10	1	52	4	5
31	8-73	3.9	29	N	50	2+	50	1.2	82	N	60	2+	45	1.8	8	N	<10	1	46	3	5
32	10-73	5.3	17	N	50	2	65	1.1	86	N	50	3	74	5.2	.5	N	20	2	50	5	3
33	11-73	5.2	29	1+	30	2+	52	1.6	108	N	60	3	70	2.4	12	N	20	2	34	3	2

semen. The cause of this condition remains a mystery. If the postcoital test is satisfactory, the viscosity is not interfering with sperm migration and no therapy is necessary. However, some of these patients have poor postcoital tests in which the semen specimen is a solid globular mass that cannot even be poured, even though the tapioca-like gel of coagulation has completely disappeared. It has been observed that there is no direct correlation between high seminal viscosity and poor motility in specimens with sperm counts of greater than 60 million per ml, but high viscosity in semen with low counts has an important adverse effect on the motility of spermatozoa. Microscopic examination may reveal that the sperm move sluggishly and even seem to vibrate in place without forward progression.[75] In general, high seminal viscosity does not in itself produce fertility problems unless it is accompanied by poor sperm motility.

Treatment to reduce seminal viscosity by such indirect measures as overhydration of the patient, prostatic massages, and administration of atropine antagonists or parenteral hyaluronidase has not been effective. However, there are several possible methods of reducing seminal viscosity which should be tried only if the postcoital test is poor. One method consists of using the first portion of the split ejaculate for insemination if the viscosity of this portion is lower than that of the entire ejaculate. In a second method the viscous specimen is transferred into a Luer-lock syringe and forcibly ejected into a glass container through an 18 or 19 gauge needle. The specimen is then poured back into the syringe, and the procedure is repeated about five times. After this treatment, the semen is no longer viscous and flows like water, with no demonstrable damage to the sperm cells themselves. The specimen is used for insemination.

Semen can also be mixed with Alevaire, a mucolytic solution, in a ratio of 1:1 by volume. Alevaire (now manufactured by Breon Laboratories, Inc.) is harmless to viable cells, and its pH is compatible with the preservation of sperm motility. As a mucolytic detergent, Alevaire is chemically inert and is highly active in reducing seminal viscosity.[1] We have found Alevaire most useful for this purpose when it is employed as a precoital douche. It is readily available in individual 60 ml. bottles, the entire contents of which are allowed to flow into the vagina through the douche nozzle. The small amount of Alevaire that remains within the vagina will effectively reduce the viscosity of the semen deposited immediately afterward during intercourse.[4] This method obviously eliminates the need for insemination and is most acceptable to patients.

Another method that does not require insemination is the prescription for the husband of a conjugated estrogen, Premarin, 1.25 mg daily for 5 days, starting with day 1 of his wife's menstrual cycle. The seminal viscosity will often be markedly reduced around midcycle 1 week later. However, estrogen can suppress pituitary gonadotropin release, and this medication should not be used by the husband for more than three consecutive cycles.

Unrewarding attempts to reduce seminal viscosity were made by adding hyaluronidase directly to the specimen *in vitro*. This will succeed only if the pH of the specimen is dropped to 6.4 or below. Unfortunately, semen is normally slightly alkaline, and when the pH is dropped to the acid range, sperm motility is halted; this method of reducing seminal viscosity is therefore of no value.

NONLIQUEFACTION OF SEMEN

Occasional semen specimens are observed in which the gel or coagulum which forms immediately after ejaculation persists, failing to liquify within the usual 5 to 20 minutes. The process of seminal coagulation is thought to be enzymatic in nature, and the substrate for the gel formation consists of a proteinlike material secreted by the seminal vesicles. Normally, after liquefaction takes place the sperm trapped in the coagulum can achieve their full motility. The seminal fluid after coagulation and liquefaction has a characteristic viscosity which may occasionally be too high, as previously noted. Viscosity is, however, a different phenomenon from coagulation,[2, 72] and the two terms should not be confused.

Bunge and Sherman[16] reported an effective method for dealing with problems of persistent delayed liquefaction of semen employing the *in vitro* addition of a 4 per cent solution of alpha-amylases in Locke's solution. They had discovered by chance that human saliva had the capability of liquefying a semen specimen brought to the laboratory for analysis. (Serendipity had a role in this discovery when a technician, frustrated in his attempts to do a sperm count on the nonliquefied specimen, asked in despair, "What should I do with this thick glob?" and received the equally desperate reply, "Spit in it!") The use of alpha-amylase solution as a precoital douche and, more recently, the use of a cocoa-butter vaginal suppository containing 50 mg. of alpha-amylase have been found effective in overcoming the nonliquefaction problem. Bunge has reported pregnancies after prescribing the intravaginal application of alpha-amylase on appropriate days of the ovarian cycle, but there is still some question as to whether nonliquefaction of semen *per se* can be a cause for infertility.[49] However, alpha-amylase may affect the vaginal or cervical secretions containing glycogen and possibly provide an energy source for spermatozoal activity.

RETROGRADE EJACULATION

The phenomenon of retrograde ejaculation, a backward ejaculation of semen into the urinary bladder, was discussed in Chapter 1 under disorders of ejaculation. Hope for fertility need not be abandoned in patients with retrograde ejaculation. The following technique for retrieval of sperm from the bladder may be employed.[6, 33]

1. Starting the day before collection, the patient alkalinizes his urine with bicarbonate of soda, 1 teaspoon in a glass of water every 4 hours.

2. In the urologist's office, the bladder is emptied by catheterization and irrigated repeatedly with Ringer's glucose solution.

3. After irrigation is completed and the bladder emptied, 2 ml. of the same solution is left in the bladder, and the catheter is removed.

4. Manually induced ejaculation is immediately performed.

5. The entire contents of the bladder are then removed by voiding or, if necessary, by reintroduction of the catheter.

The specimen thus retrieved is centrifuged to obtain 1 ml. of concentrated sediment. This often contains motile sperm in good concentration and may be used for direct insemination of the wife. It is important to keep the sperm in an alkaline medium, because acidification will result in the loss of sperm motility. Many successful pregnancies have resulted from this technique.

Recent studies have suggested a new medical approach to the management of men who are infertile because of retrograde ejaculation secondary to neuropathic failure of the bladder neck to close during ejaculation. Retrograde ejaculation in some patients with diabetic neuropathy can be corrected by the oral administration of a sympathomimetic drug, phenylpropanolamine (Ornade), 1 spansule twice daily.[70]

Alternatively, brompheniramine (Dimetane) a drug with antihistaminic and anticholinergic properties, also successfully corrects retrograde ejaculation in some diabetic males. Disappointingly, at this writing no pregnancies have been reported with either drug.

Retrograde ejaculation in one man who had undergone unilateral orchiectomy and retroperitoneal lymphadenectomy for a malignant testicular tumor was reversed by the repeated intravenous administration of synephrine, an alpha-adrenergic drug.[71] In five other patients with aspermia, this drug produced no ejaculation, presumably because the problem was cessation of contraction of the seminal vesicles and vas following the retroperitoneal dissection rather than the previously supposed retrograde ejaculation.[37]

Surgical correction of bladder neck obstructions utilizing Y–V plasty can lead to retrograde ejaculation owing to surgically induced incompetence of the internal sphincter at the bladder neck. A reconstructive transvesical surgical procedure was described in 1975 by Abrahams and Waterhouse.[1] They employed it in two patients—one 36 years old and the other 24—who had presented with the problem of sterility secondary to retrograde ejaculation. These patients had undergone Y–V plasties for bladder neck obstruction 8 and 4 years earlier, respectively, and both had cystograms that showed contrast material in the posterior urethra, indicating that the bladder neck was wide open in the resting state. In the reconstructive transvesical operation, the bladder neck is closed and the internal sphincter is restored to the diameter of a No. 16 French Foley catheter, which is removed on the twenty-first postoperative day (Fig. 10–1).

Both patients reported the re-establishment of normal antegrade ejaculation by the fourth week after surgery, and one has fathered a child.

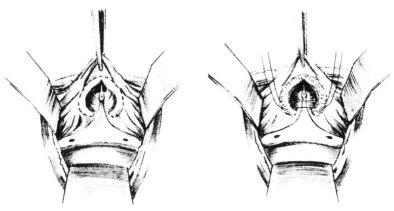

An inverted figure "U" is fashioned.   Both its limbs are sutured together.

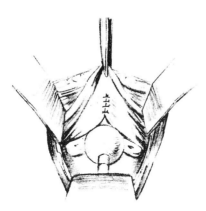

The internal sphincter is then rebuilt.

Figure 10–1. The Abrahams-Waterhouse operation for closure of the bladder neck.

FREEZING SPERM

Spectacular success has been achieved in the field of animal husbandry with the use of frozen semen. The important scientific and practical advances resulting from the use of frozen dairy bull semen are attributable to the development of effective methods of diluting bull semen without loss of fertility. After freezing and storing the diluted semen, it is possible to inseminate successfully a large number of cows with the sperm from the single ejaculate of a prize bull.

The application of the freezing technique to human sperm has been reviewed by J. K. Sherman.[66] Spallanzini in 1776 was perhaps the first to report observations on the effects of freezing temperatures on human spermatozoa, and Montegazza in 1866 was the first to suggest banks for frozen human sperm. During the period 1938 to 1945, it was observed that some human spermatozoa could survive freezing and storage at temperatures as low as minus 269°C. Much effort has been expended on devising methods of improving the survival of motile sperm during the process of freezing, storing, and thawing human semen. Research has been directed at evaluating such factors as the rate of cooling and rewarming, length of time stored at the maintenance temperature, and pretreatment with protective substances (e.g., glycerol, dimethyl sulfoxide, and diluents).[24]

Human spermatozoa frozen with nitrogen vapor and stored at minus 196°C. have retained their motility and fertilizing capacity during prolonged periods,[65] and normal births following impregnation with these sperm have occurred after 10 years of storage.[39] The nitrogen-vapor method of freezing does seem to permit a greater percentage of motile cells to survive freezing and thawing, but it is still in the realm of science fiction to believe that this technique has wide application to the management of infertility in the oligospermic male with poor sperm motility. A semen specimen with good initial motility is required if fertilizing potential after freezing is to be retained. The process of freezing, storing, concentrating, and inseminating the preserved multiple ejaculates of oligospermic men whose semen has poor sperm motility is, for practical purposes, beyond reach with present techniques because freeze-thawing can only further impair the motility of the spermatozoa. Behrman and Sawada[11] reported no success in achieving pregnancy using frozen semen with poor sperm motility; in their study six to eight specimens from each husband were collected, concentrated, and stored. Rubin et al.[56] emphasize that poor semen freezes and thaws poorly, resulting in increased loss in sperm motility; they conclude that freeze-preservation of pathologic semen from oligospermic men is not feasible. The suggestion by the proprietors of commercial sperm-freezing banks that such poor specimens can be treated and used to produce pregnancies is to be condemned as the worst sort of hucksterism, taking cruel advantage of the infertile couples' desperate desire for children.

Much is still unknown about the freeze-preservation of human sperm. In the many pregnancies that have already resulted from frozen donor semen the newborn appear to be at least the equals of their controls both physically and mentally.[77] The state of their future health and reproductive propensities remain to be established. However, studies on DNA of sperm after long periods of storage indicate no detectable biochemical changes.[13, 67] The results of experience in animal husbandry, numbering literally in the millions, tend to mollify anxiety on this score.

Although the feasibility of freeze-preservation of human sperm has been established, it is clear that *storage of fertile semen does not guarantee future fertility*. Beck and Silverstein[10] reported a wide range of motility after thawing among donors of proven fertility (15 to 45 per cent) and demonstrated that motility prior to freezing, paternity history, or both are no guarantee of sperm viability after the semen has been frozen. This must give pause to the use of sperm banks as "fertility insurance" for men undergoing vasectomy who wish to preserve their semen for future impregnation if there is a change of mind after sterilization. A trial specimen submitted to freezing and thawing is suggested for any man contemplating such "fertility insurance." Behrman[13] suggests that there may be some inherent genetic weakness in some human sperm specimens, a weakness which is susceptible to freezing procedures as carried out at this time. He poses the following immediate research questions: (1) Why is fertility reduced by freeze storage? (2) What is the nature of the change during freezing at the molecular level? (3) What is the ideal vehicle or medium for protection during freezing? (4) What changes are required in the technique of freezing? (5) What criteria should we use to judge the fertilizing capacity of any given specimen?

Because at the present time, sperm motility is lost in the process of freezing and thawing, it is emphasized that the therapeutic use of this technique for the *infertile* male is still a tool to be perfected.

Future eugenic applications of the storage of frozen ejaculates,[50] once the subject of science fiction, now appear to be possible. By storing his ejaculate, a man can induce conception in the absence of testes, in old age, and long after his death. Thus the reproductive effectiveness of husband or desirable donor can be extended indefinitely.[66] For example, a patient with a neoplasm requiring therapy with radiation or cytotoxic drugs that will impair his fertility, or a patient faced with surgery that might impair the ejaculation process can have his ejaculates collected and preserved prior to therapy, thereby providing potential fertility via insemination at a later date.

MALE SEXUAL DYSFUNCTION

The role of sexuality in human fertility is obvious, yet it is all too often overlooked by the physician.[19] In a 5-year study of the causative factors in 1294 consecutive cases of male infertility in one large practice from 1965 to 1970, sexual problems were the primary cause of the couples' infertility in 5.5 per cent of cases.[18] If our added total experience is considered, male sexual dysfunction may now be the primary causative factor or an important contributing factor in almost 10 per cent of involuntarily infertile marriages, especially when it is remembered that a number of men have sexual problems as well as oligospermia. Thus, the sexual and psychological problems of infertility are highly important. Even in those cases in which there is a clear-cut organic cause, psychological repercussions are inevitable by the mere revelation of the existence of infertility in the male. Furthermore, the diagnostic tests and treatments themselves may create psychological difficulties. Tolstoy has written that "Man survives earthquakes, epidemics, the horrors of disease and all the agonies of the soul, but for all time his most tormenting tragedy has been, is and will be—the tragedy of the bedroom."[55]

SEXUAL HISTORY

The importance of eliciting a meticulous and thorough sexual history cannot be overemphasized. There is no area in medicine where more tact, sympathy, and understanding are required than in eliciting a sexual history. It must be done by a physician with a caring and nonjudgmental attitude in a *relaxed,* confidential, private office setting. There is room for only one nervous person in a physician's office at one time, and this is particularly true in sexual data gathering.

One easy method of taking a sexual history, is chronological and general, the questions slowly leading to those that may elicit more anxiety, such as queries relating to homosexuality. But the questions must be asked, because the patient with sexual problems seldom volunteers information about inadequacy. Written questionnaires may be helpful, especially if they are answered by both husband and wife, but they hardly substitute for a clinical interview in eliciting information that will be helpful in the solution of the problem. No standard form of interview will ever suffice, and it must always be tailored to the sophistication and comfort of the patient. Moreover, this interview can also relieve anxiety and be therapeutic for the patient, since it gives the physician the opportunity to dispel misinformation and to give reassurance about the general normalcy of many forms of sexual behavior that may have caused shame or were felt by the patient to be perverse and unique to him. The physician should allow time at the end of the interview for the patient's questions or for emphasis of important points.

PSYCHOGENIC IMPOTENCE

In the wide spectrum of sexual problems, the urologist is most frequently called upon to deal with the impotent male, and at least 90 per cent of these problems will fall into the area of psychogenic impotence.[32, 47, 48] Walker has reviewed some of the psychological conditions that interfere with a man's ability to ejaculate into the depth of the vagina.[74] Psychogenic causes may be responsible for (1) simple inability to have an erection, (2) partial or weak erections, (3) inability to sustain an erection long enough to penetrate, (4) orgasm before or right after entry, and (5) ejaculatory incompetency—the inability to ejaculate during vaginal containment.

The literature on impotence in sexologic, urologic, and gynecologic journals strikingly underplays the role of depression. This common malady with its protean symptoms rarely exists without some form of impotence. Rapid diagnosis and treatment of depression, should be instituted in all cases when necessary, before further work-up or treatment is undertaken. Neurotic depressions properly and promptly treated have an excellent prognosis. Serious psychiatric disorders such as schizophrenia or manic depressive psychoses, or even a serious question of these diagnoses, should prompt psychiatric consultation without further work-ups which might add too much strain to an already overloaded psyche.

There are many types of impotence, but from the point of view of *fertility*, impotence may be defined as the inability to have satisfactory erection and discharge of the ejaculate into the vagina at the desired time of the wife's menstrual cycle. The causes of impotence may be organic or psychogenic. Penile erection depends not only upon structural neuromuscular and vascular components but also to a large extent upon the emotional state of the individual. By far the most frequent cause of impotence is psychogenic factors.

Psychogenic impotence is generally selective in nature—it occurs under one set of circumstances but not under another, e.g., a man may be impotent with his wife but with no one else, or he may be able to masturbate to ejaculation but be unable to penetrate a vagina. If a man is capable of ejaculating by masturbation or by nocturnal emissions it can be stated with assurance that there is no physical factor preventing intravaginal ejaculations.

It is important to note, however, that although psychogenic impotence is usually selective in nature, it is not selective if it is produced by depression or chronic drug abuse.[74] The most popular and prevalent social drug abuse problem is alcoholism. This is becoming prevalent in a younger and younger group of men and eventually leads to impotence. Because alcohol is accepted socially and legally it is a frequently overlooked culprit.

The common problem of premature ejaculation can be handled better by the counseling physician by such methods as the "squeeze technique"[48] than by exploratory psychotherapy. At the other extreme, ejaculatory incompetence is a very severe and refractory malady. Walker cites four cases of primary ejaculatory incompetence, men who have never experienced an orgasm in any situation.[74] All were men in their twenties. Three of the four were married, and all were rigidly controlling, obsessive-compulsive men. They had been examined urologically and were found to have no physical problems. These cases were refractory to exploratory and behavioral psychotherapy as well as to attempts to produce ejaculation with the electrovibrator even while under the influence of sodium amytal.

Treatment of the psychologic sexual problems of infertility is difficult but rewarding. It is to the credit, not of traditional analytic psychiatry, which has its roots in sexual theory, but of behavioral psychology, gynecology, and urology that we owe our knowledge of sexual problems. Some problems such as deep depression or serious psychological illnesses should prompt a psychiatric consultation, but the vast majority of sexual problems can be handled by the understanding urologist, internist, or gynecologist.

If the patient does not have a severe psychogenic disturbance he will often respond well to simple measures of reassurance and instruction. It should be emphasized that a previous poor sexual performance need not preclude satisfactory coitus the next time. The patient should be made aware that he is in a stressful situation and, because the demands on his body are greater, he needs a good diet and healthy exercise.

In some patients with poor erections, the administration of human chorionic gonadotropin (HCG), 4000 units twice weekly for 4 to 6 weeks, combined with supportive counselling will result in improved sexual performance and pregnancy.[19] The temporary increase in endogenous androgen production by the testes and the supportive reassurance will often be enough to cure the vicious circle of problems relating to psychogenic impotence, particularly problems with secondary erectile impotence and those with premature ejaculation.

Infrequent sexual activity causes infertility problems in some couples.[19] Sometimes libido is at a low level, and coitus may occur once a month or less. These couples often seem to repress awareness of this fact and express surprise when it is discussed with them. Of 19 couples whose infertility was caused by infrequency of coitus, divorce occurred in two cases. Encouragement resulted in increased sexual frequency and pregnancy in nine couples, and stimulation of the husband with human chorionic gonadotropin (4000 units twice weekly for 6 weeks) was used successfully in six additional couples.

On the other hand, some men have good semen specimens but ejaculate with such high frequency that they often deposit specimens of poor quality at the time of coitus.[23] In one such case the patient had coitus with his wife and other women and averaged 18 ejaculations per week. The problem in five other cases was excessive masturbation that resulted in up to five ejaculations daily. These cases responded to counselling and psychologic help.[19]

Mention should also be made of couples in whom actual coitus never took place, and the wives had intact hymens. Yet these couples were puzzled as to why there was no pregnancy! It seems inconceivable that such lack of knowledge of sexuality can exist today, but it again emphasizes the need to investigate even the most obvious possible causes.

ORGANIC IMPOTENCE

Organic impotence is the loss of the ability to initiate, sustain, or successfully conclude the act of coitus because certain physiologic processes affecting the vascular and neuromuscular components have been disturbed. A common cause of organic impotence is diabetes with its vascular and neuropathic sequelae. Indeed, erectile impotence is the presenting symptom in about 10 per cent of diabetic males; it can often be helped by medical management of the diabetes early in the course of the disease.[21] Retrograde ejaculation may occur as a sequela of diabetic neuropathy but is not helped by medical control of the diabetes. In the diabetic male, retrograde ejaculation may be a precursor of total ejaculatory impotence, and again, this problem cannot be corrected by careful treatment and control of the diabetes itself.[5] It may be well to advise married diabetic males who desire to have children to start their families as soon as possible to avoid the potential problems with ejaculation that may occur later in the course of the disease.

Arteriosclerotic vascular disease, which may be either pronounced, as in the case of LeRiche's syndrome of thrombosis at the aortic bifurcation, or a less severe vascular insufficiency, may be a cause of organic impotence. Vascular conditions with a high or normal blood flow rate are not associated with impaired potency, whereas depressed blood flow rates, as in arterial insufficiency, are found with impotence.[51, 52] A low penile blood pressure in impotent patients indicates an obstruction of the blood flow in the main vessels supplying the penis, although other evidence of peripheral vascular disease may be minimal.[25, 44] Although impotence is thus a known symptom of arteriosclerotic disease of the aorta and iliac vessels, surgery such as aortoiliac reconstruction is more likely to cause further disturbance in sexual function than the disease. Many men find that they have developed ejaculatory failure after the operation, although erection can be achieved. The ability to achieve penile erection depends both on the volume of blood flowing into the internal iliac arteries and on the integrity of the pelvic splanchnic nerves. Ejaculation depends on the sympathetic nerves, particularly those in the superior hypogastric plexus lying in front of the aortic bifurcation. It has been suggested that the vascular surgeon should preserve the superior hypogastric sympathetic plexus (presacral nerve) during endarterectomy or aortoiliac reconstruction and that only the sympathetic nerves on the right side that supply the superior hypogastric plexus should be divided; those on the left should be preserved, and the sympathetic nerves from the lumbar chain on the left side of the aorta should also be kept intact. This maneuver by the vascular surgeon can preserve both erectile and ejaculatory sexual function in at least 90 per cent of patients whose impotence is due to arteriosclerotic disease of the aorta and iliac vessels.[57]

Priapism may be a sequela of a variety of diseases, or it may be idiopathic. Long-standing priapism is almost always succeeded by impotence. The postpriapic patient has normal penile sensation and ejaculatory reflexes but may be impotent because his penis is limp. He cannot obtain an erection because of the disruption of the vascular supply mechanism. To prevent this disruption from reaching the irreversible stage, both the corpus spongiosum[58] and the saphenous vein[28] have been utilized to achieve an alternative pathway for venous drainage in patients with priapism.

Erectile impotence can follow spinal cord injury or trauma such as "straddle" injury to the perineum with damage to the perineal nerves, accidental rupture of the corpora of the erect penis, or pelvic fracture with neurologic injury. Perineal nerve injury during perineal prostatectomy can also be a cause. Lumbar sympathectomy can interfere with venous pathways for erection and ejaculation, as can damage to the nerve supply during pelvic or retroperitoneal surgery.[37]

Neurologic diseases with myelopathy or peripheral neuropathy can result in impotence. Lumbar disc disease[63] can cause impotence, but surgical correction of the disc pressure can restore potency.

Such endocrinologic disorders as primary or secondary hypogonadism and metabolic disorders that result in renal failure can lead to true organic impotence,[59, 64, 73] but in these there may be concomitant loss of libido, as in the heroin or morphine addict.

However, in many patients with organic impotence not due to debilitating disease or severe endocrinologic or metabolic derangement, and especially in the age group with which we are dealing, the libido remains intact, and the loss of ability to achieve an erection is extremely distressing to the patient. External splints, so-called "coital training devices"[43] have been applied to the limp penis to give it an outer skeleton of support, but these are largely unsatisfactory both to the patient and to his sexual partner.

Proper management requires that each case be considered individually and that all possible etiologic factors be evaluated before making therapeutic recommendations. Some patients with organic impotence will not respond to appropriate therapy, or their anatomic lesions will prove to be untreatable. In these patients an implantable penile prosthesis may be used to facilitate coitus, even if ejaculation cannot be achieved.[14, 26, 40, 53, 62, 68]

We encounter many patients with hypertension or cardiac irregularities who have developed problems with potency and ejaculation from the use of such sympathetic blocking agents as guanethidine or Inderal, which should be avoided if possible. Other satisfactory therapeutic agents which will not subject the patient to the added strain of sexual dysfunction are available; one such antihypertensive drug is clonidine hydrochloride (Catapres).

SEMEN SPECIMEN COLLECTION USING THE ELECTROVIBRATOR

In many cases of ejaculatory impotence, in which the patient has good erections but is unable to produce ejaculation, even through masturbation,

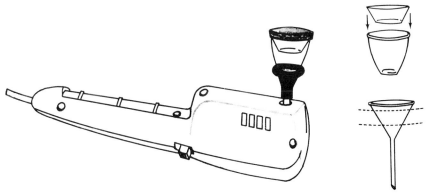

Figure 10–2. Diagram illustrating the modification of the electrovibrator for use in the induction of ejaculation for semen collection.

we have been successful in obtaining ejaculates for insemination by the use of a simple electrovibrator,[60, 69] which is fitted with a collection cup and applied to the glans penis before the appartus is turned on. The pulsatile vibrations are applied directly to the glans. The use of the electrovibrator eliminates the need for uncomfortable electric shocks through a rectal electrode as used by some workers. Some patients with neurogenic or psychogenic ejaculatory impotence have delivered semen specimens by this technique, and it is worth trying.

We have employed either the "duo massage" vibrator model manufactured by the Oster Company, Milwaukee, Wisconsin or the General Electric hand vibrator. The vibrator can be adapted for the purpose of semen collection by fitting a collection beaker into the rubber cup attachment supplied with the vibrator (Fig. 10–2).

The semen collection beaker for use with the vibrator is fashioned from a No. 7913 Vycor 50-ml. beaker with a 1-inch base and a 2-inch mouth, obtainable from a scientific supply house. A trap is provided by fitting the wide portion of a 2-inch plastic funnel (the narrow portion and stem of which have been cut off) into the mouth of the beaker and taping around the edge to secure it in place.

ARTIFICIAL INSEMINATION WITH THE HUSBAND'S SEMEN

In dealing with the infertile couple the urologist and the gynecologist can effectively combine their talents in selecting patients for, and perfecting techniques of, AIH (artificial insemination with semen obtained from the husband). The actual process of insemination is usually in the province of the gynecologist, for the procedure must be timed to coincide with ovulation. It has been suggested that more homologous inseminations be performed if the semen volume is 1.5 ml. or less[49] and if the semen quality is otherwise good and the results of the postcoital test are poor, as the low volume in itself may be a factor in infertility by not allowing adequate access of the sperm to the cervical mucus.

Again, when semen quality is borderline, with less than optimal sperm concentration or sperm motility, insemination with the husband's sperm may increase the chances for a pregnancy. When the semen volume is 3 ml. or more, semen analysis on the split ejaculate is worthwhile; only the better fraction of the split ejaculate should be used for insemination.[3, 22] It is emphasized that in only 90 per cent of instances will the first part of the split ejaculate be found to have the higher concentration of sperm. The specimen must therefore be checked first—it cannot just be assumed that the first portion is the better part. Occasionally, insemination with the second fraction will be indicated.[4]

Recent research on the in vitro stimulation of sperm by caffeine[61] indicates that both the per cent of motility and the grade of forward progression of ejaculated human spermatozoa can be increased significantly and maintained by the addition of a buffered solution containing 6 millimoles of caffeine. The mechanism of action of caffeine on spermatozoan motility is still not clear. We do know that caffeine inhibits cyclic nucleotide phosphodiesterases—enzymes that are involved in human spermatozoan glycolysis, although the mechanism of caffeine inhibition is not completely known. In the light of these findings, it is possible that caffeine added to semen could help to improve the fertility of patients whose specimens show low sperm motility. Artificial insemination of specimens treated with caffeine and the use of a precoital caffeine douche by the wives of these patients are currently under investigation.

Another area of current research involves the elimination of sperm-agglutinating and sperm-immobilizing antibodies by washing the sperm and then resuspending them in normal acellular seminal plasma.[34] Filtration of whole semen with millipore filters (pore size 0.45 m) removes all spermatozoa and yields sperm-free seminal plasma. The washed sperm can then be resuspended in the normal sperm-free seminal plasma and used for insemination. This procedure is still in the experimental stage and cannot yet be considered the solution to problems of sperm autoantibodies.

Impotent patients who are unable to ejaculate into the vagina at the proper time of the cycle but can masturbate can produce semen specimens which can be used for AIH. In some patients with psychogenic impotence and in paraplegic patients, the electrovibrator can be used to obtain the semen specimen for AIH.

An occasional impotent patient who can ejaculate only during nocturnal emissions can wear a Milex sheath during his sleep and catch the ejaculate in the sheath. He can be taught to use his own semen to inseminate his wife. This circumstance occurs only rarely but the technique does offer a possible solution. It was used successfully in the case of an orthodox Jewish couple who could not allow insemination by a doctor but desperately desired a child.

Severe hypospadias, in which the urethral opening is too far from the end of the penis to permit coital intravaginal sperm deposition, is another indication for AIH.

In some cases when the husband must be away from home for long periods of time, as in the case of mariners or military personnel, good semen specimens can be frozen and preserved for insemination at the fertile time of the wife's cycle.

Rarely, when the husband has oligospermia but good sperm motility, the specimen can be frozen and concentrated to provide a better chance for insemination,[66] but the infertile husband who has a combination of low sperm count and excellent sperm motility is indeed exceptional. This freezing technique should not be used for concentrating oligospermic specimens with *poor* motility because motility, in the thawed concentrate will be even worse.

RELIGIOUS PROSCRIPTIONS AND INFERTILITY PRACTICE

The devout Catholic patient cannot masturbate for semen collection but can have intercourse while wearing a perforated condom. The ordinary condom cannot be employed for the collection of a semen specimen because the sperm-immobilizing properties of the materials used in its manufacture will interfere with any evaluation of sperm motility. A suitable technique for collecting semen from Catholic patients is discussed in Chapter 5.

The orthodox Jew may present a more difficult problem than the Catholic when collection of a semen specimen is necessary. Although masturbation is not acceptable to strictly orthodox Jewish patients, coitus interruptus and ejaculation directly into a collection bottle, or the use of a Milex sheath during intercourse is acceptable to most Rabbinic authorities. It is definitely not necessary to pierce a hole in the sheath (as for Catholic patients), so there will be no problem in collecting the entire specimen in the sheath or losing any of the sample during collection. These semen collection methods have been sanctioned by Rabbinic authorities, and it is not necessary to obtain the semen specimen by spooning it from the vagina after intercourse as is commonly believed. There are occasional orthodox patients who will not collect a semen specimen under any circumstances, and for these a postcoital test may be of value, as discussed in Chapter 5.

The physician dealing with fertility problems may find himself confronted by problems in evaluating and treating infertility in orthodox Jewish couples because of their strict adherence to Jewish law. Jewish law poses obstacles in semen collection, genital surgery, management of menstrual problems, and homologous (AIH) and donor (AID) insemination. Guidelines which will be acceptable to most orthodox Jewish patients have been published. These guidelines allow the observance of ritual laws and still permit evaluation and therapy from the standpoint of the infertility specialist.[27]

REFERENCES

1. Abrahams, J. I., Solish, G. I., Boorjian, P. C. and Waterhouse, R. K.: Surgical correction of retrograde ejaculation. J. Urol., *114*:888, 1975.
1A. Amelar, R. D.: The use of Alevaire in the routine study of sperm morphology. Fertil. Steril., *7*:346, 1956.
2. Amelar, R. D.: Coagulation, liquefaction and viscosity of human semen. J. Urol., *87*:187, 1962.
3. Amelar, R. D. and Hotchkiss, R. S.: The split ejaculate: its use in the management of male infertility. Fertil. Steril., *16*:46, 1965.
4. Amelar, R. D.: Infertility in Men: Diagnosis and Treatment. Philadelphia, F. A. Davis Co., 1966.
5. Amelar, R. D. and Dubin, L.: Infertility in the Male. *In* Practice of Surgery. Vol. 2, Urology. Hagerstown, Maryland, Harper and Row, 1971.
6. Amelar, R. D. and Dubin, L.: Male infertility: Current diagnosis and treatment. Urology, *1*:1, 1973.
7. Amelar, R. D., Dubin, L. and Schoenfeld, C.: Semen analysis: An office technique. Urology, *2*:605, 1973.
8. Amelar, R. D. and Dubin, L.: A coital technique for the promotion of fertility. Urology, *5*:228, 1975.
9. Andaloro, V. A. and Dube, A.: Treatment of retrograde ejaculation with brompheniramine (Dimetane). Urology, *5*:520, 1975.
10. Beck, W. W., Jr. and Silverstein, I.: Variable motility recovery of spermatozoa after freeze preservation. Fertil. Steril., *26*:212, 1975 (abstract).
11. Behrman, .S. J. and Sawada, Y.: Heterologous and homologous insemination with human semen frozen and stored in a liquid nitrogen refrigeration. Fertil. Steril., *17*:457, 1966.
12. Behrman, S. J. and Kistner, R. W.: Progress in Infertility, 2d ed. Boston, Little, Brown and Co., 1975, p. 786.
13. Behrman, S. J.: Editorial: The preservation of semen. Fertil. Steril., *24*:396, 1973.
14. Bias, H. I., Leverett, C. L., Parry, W. L. and Halverstadt, D. B.: Implantable penile prostheses in impotent males. Urology, *5*:224, 1975.
15. Budd, H. A., Jr.: Brompheniramine (Dimetane) in treatment of retrograde ejaculation. Urology, *6*:131, 1975.
16. Bunge, R. G. and Sherman, J. K.: Liquefaction of human semen by alpha amylase. Fertil. Steril., *5*:353, 1954.
17. Bunge, R. D.: Some observations on the male ejaculate. Fertil. Steril., *21*:639, 1970.
18. Dubin, L. and Amelar, R. D.: Etiologic factors in 1294 consecutive cases of male infertility. Fertil. Steril., *22*:469, 1971.
19. Dubin, L. and Amelar, R. D.: Sexual causes of male infertility. Fertil. Steril., *23*:579, 1972.
20. Eliason, R. and Lindholmer, C.: Distribution and properties of spermatozoa in different fractions of split ejaculates. Fertil. Steril., *23*:252, 1972.
21. Ellenberg, M.: Impotence in diabetes: Neurologic factors. Ann. Intern. Med., *75*:213, 1971.
22. Farris, E. J. and Murphy, D. P.: The characteristics of the two parts of the partitioned ejaculate and the advantages of its use for intrauterine insemination. Fertil. Steril., *11*:465, 1960.

23. Freund, M.: Effect of frequency of emission on semen output and on estimate of daily sperm production in man. J. Reprod. Fertil., 6:269, 1963.
24. Freund, M. and Wiederman, J.: Factors affecting the dilution, freezing and storage of human semen. J. Reprod. Fertil., 11:1, 1966.
25. Gaskell, P.: Importance of penile blood pressure in cases of impotence. Canad. Med. Assoc. J., 105:1047, 1971.
26. Gee, W. F.: A history of the surgical treatment of impotence. Urology, 5:401, 1975.
27. Gordon, J. A., Amelar, R. D., Dubin, L. and Tendler, M. D.: Infertility practice and Orthodox Jewish Law. Fertil. Steril., 26:480, 1975.
28. Grayhack, J. T., McCullough, W., O'Connor, V., Jr. and Trippel, O.: Venous bypass to control priapism. Invest. Urol., 1:509, 1964.
29. Greene, L. F., Kelalis, P. P. and Weeks, R. E.: Retrograde ejaculation of semen due to diabetic neuropathy. Fertil. Steril., 14:617, 1963.
30. Hartman, C. G.: Science and the Safe Period: A Compendium of Human Reproduction. Baltimore, The Williams & Wilkins Co., 1962, pp. 64–74.
31. Harvey, C.: The use of partitioned ejaculates in investigating the role of accessory secretions in human semen. Studies on Fertility, Proc. Soc. Stud. Fertil., 8:3, 1956.
32. Hastings, D. W.: Impotence and Frigidity. Boston, Little, Brown and Co., 1963.
33. Hotchkiss, R. S., Pinto, A. B. and Kleegman, S. J.: Artificial insemination with semen recovered from the bladder. Fertil. Steril., 6:37, 1955.
34. Jecht, E. W. and Poon, C. H.: Preparation of sperm-free seminal plasma from human semen. Fertil. Steril., 26:1, 1975.
35. Johnson, T. H.: A simple technique for direct semen examination. J. Urol., 89:262, 1963.
36. Kaplan, H. S.: The New Sex Therapy. New York, Brunner-Mazel, Inc., 1974.
37. Kedia, K. R., Markland, C. and Fraley, E. E.: Sexual function following high retroperitoneal lymphadenectomy. J. Urol., 114:237, 1975.
38. Kleegman, S. J. and Kaufman, S. A.: Infertility in Women. Philadelphia, F. A. Davis Co., 1966.
39. Kleegman, S., Amelar, R. D., Sherman, J. K., Hirschhorn, K. and Pilpel, H.: Roundtable: Artificial donor insemination. Med. Aspects Human Sex., 4:85, 1970.
40. Kothari, D. R., Timm, G. W., Frohib, D. A. and Bradley, W. E.: An implantable fluid transfer system for treatment of impotence. J. Biomech., 5:567, 1972.
41. Lardy, H. A., Ghosh, D. and Plaut, G. W. E.: A metabolic regulator in mammalian spermatozoa. Science, 109:365, 1949.
42. Lindholmer, C.: Survival of human spermatozoa in different fractions of split ejaculate. Fertil. Steril., 24:521, 1973.
43. Lowenstein, J.: Treatment of impotence: A coitus training apparatus. Brit. Med. J., 2:49, 1941.
44. Malvar, T., Baron, T. and Clark, S. S.: Assessment of potency with the Doppler flowmeter. Urology, 2:396, 1973.
45. Mann, T., Short, R. V., Walton, A., Archer, R. K., and Miller, W. C.: The "tail end sample" of stallion semen. J. Agricult. Sci., 49:301, 1957.
46. Mann, T.: The Biochemistry of Semen and of the Male Reproductive Tract. New York, John Wiley & Sons, Inc., 1964, pp. 107–112.
47. Masters, W. H. and Johnson, V. E.: Human Sexual Response. Boston, Little, Brown and Co., 1966.
48. Masters, W. H. and Johnson, V. E.: Human Sexual Inadequacy. Boston, Little, Brown and Co., 1970.
49. McLane, C. M.: Symposium on Infertility (Foreword). Clin. Obs. Gynecol., 8:11, 1965.
50. Muller, H. J.: Genetic progress by voluntarily conducted germinal choice. In Wolstenholme, G. (ed.): Man and His Future. Boston, Little, Brown and Co., 1963.
51. Newman, H. F., Northrop, J. D. and Devlen, J.: Mechanisms of human penile erection. J. Invest. Urol., 1:350, 1964.
52. Newman, H. F.: Vibratory sensitivity of the penis. Fertil. Steril., 21:791, 1970.
53. Pearman, R.: Insertion of a Silastic penile prosthesis for the treatment of organic sexual impotence. J. Urol., 107:802, 1972.
54. Pedron, N., Giner, J., Hicks, J. J. and Rosado, A.: Comparative glycolytic metabolism in normal and oligoasthenospermic subjects. Fertil. Steril., 26:309, 1975.
55. Pumpian-Mindlin, E.: Contributions of psychoanalytic theory to the understanding of sexual development and behavior. In Wahl, C. W. (ed.): Sexual Problems, Diagnosis and Treatment in Medical Practice. New York, The Free Press, Macmillan Co., 1967.

56. Rubin, S. O., Anderson, L. and Boström, K.: Deep freeze preservation of normal and pathologic human semen. Scandinav. J. Urol. Nephrol., *3*:144, 1969.
57. Sabri, S. and Cotton, L. T.: Sexual function following aortoiliac reconstruction. Lancet, *2*:1218, 1971.
58. Sacher, E. C., Sayegh, E., Frensilli, F., Crum, P. and Akers, R.: Cavernospongiosium shunt in treatment of priapism. J. Urol., *108*:97, 1972.
59. Salvatierra, O., Jr., Fortzmann, J. L. and Belzer, F. O.: Sexual function in males before and after renal transplantation. Urology, *5*:64, 1975.
60. Schellen, T.: Induction of ejaculation by electrovibrator. Fertil. Steril., *19*:566, 1968.
61. Schoenfeld, C., Amelar, R. D. and Dubin, L.: Stimulation of ejaculated human spermatozoa by caffeine. Fertil. Steril., *26*:158, 1975.
62. Scott, E. B., Bradley, W. E. and Timm, G. W.: Management of erectile impotence. Urology, *2*:80, 1973.
63. Shafer, N. and Rosenblum, J.: Occult lumbar disc causing impotency. N. Y. State J. Med., *69*:2465, 1969.
64. Sherman, F. P.: Impotence in patients with chronic renal failure and dialysis: Its frequency and etiology. Fertil. Steril., *26*:221, 1975.
65. Sherman, J. K.: Long-term cryopreservation of motility and fertility of human spermatozoa. Cryobiology, *9*:332, 1972.
66. Sherman, J. K.: Synopsis of the use of frozen human semen since 1964: State of the art of human semen banking. Fertil. Steril., *24*:397, 1973.
67. Sherman, J. K. and Char, F.: Stability of Y-chromosome fluoresence during freeze-thawing and frozen storage of human spermatozoa. Fertil. Steril., *25*:311, 1974.
68. Small, M. P., Carrion, H. M. and Gordon, J. A.: Small-Carrion penile prosthesis: A new implant for management of impotence. Urology, *5*:479, 1975.
69. Sobrero, A. J., Stearns, H. E. and Blair, J. H.: Technic for the induction of ejaculation in humans. Fertil. Steril., *16*:765, 1965.
70. Stewart, B. H. and Berant, J. A.: Correction of retrograde ejaculation by sympathomimetric medication; preliminary report. Fertil. Steril., *25*:1073, 1974.
71. Stockamp, K., Schreiter, F. and Altwein, J. E.: Alpha-adrenergic drugs in retrograde ejaculation. Fertil. Steril., *25*:817, 1974.
72. Tauber, P. F. and Zaneveld, L. J. D.: Coagulation and liquefaction of human semen. *In* Hafez, E. S. E. (ed.): Human Semen and Fertility Regulation in Men. St. Louis, C. V. Mosby Co., 1976, pp. 153–166.
73. Thurm, J.: Sexual potency of patients on chronic hemodialysis. Urology, *5*:60, 1975.
74. Walker, H.: Sexual and psychological problems and infertility. *In* Proceedings of the W. W. Scott Symposium on Current Concepts in Male Infertility. University of Rochester Medical Center, April 22-24, 1976 (in press).
75. Tjioe, D. Y. and Oentoeng, S.: The viscosity of human semen and the percentage of motile spermatozoa. Fertil. Steril., *19*:562, 1968.
76. Tyler, E. T.: Sterility. New York, McGraw-Hill Book Co., 1961.
77. Tyler, E. T.: The clinical use of frozen semen banks. Fertil. Steril., *24*:413, 1973.

Chapter *11*

SURGERY FOR MALE INFERTILITY

Lawrence Dubin, M.D.
Richard D. Amelar, M.D.

Surgery is the treatment of choice in many cases of male infertility. The most important of these are described in this chapter. Varicocelectomy and testicular biopsy are discussed in Chapters 3 and 8 respectively.

PREVENTION OF INFERTILITY

Surgical measures may be used to prevent male infertility by preservation of testicular tissue. Such measures should be considered by all physicians who have patients with testicular and spermatic cord trauma, torsion of the testis, and cryptorchism.

TRAUMA TO THE TESTES

Trauma to the testes is common. Because the testicles are mobile and are protected by the tunica vaginalis, they therefore usually escape severe injury. It is rare to find a man who has not suffered some trauma to this vital area, yet significant damage is uncommon. Trauma certainly occurs more often in times of warfare, and much of our experience has been derived from reports related to it.[24, 66] Automobile and bicycle accidents as well as muggings are other contemporary causes of trauma.

IATROGENIC

Iatrogenic injuries of the spermatic cord and vas deferens at the time of hernioplasty or orchiopexy are to be avoided. Surgery in infants and children should be carried out with meticulous care since the structures involved are so small. We have successfully repaired several vasa which were ligated at the time of hernioplasty in childhood, but adequate care at the time of the original surgery would have made this unnecessary.

Iatrogenic injury by inadvertent incision of the epididymis at the time of testicular biopsy should be avoided since the epididymis, a solitary tube, will be scarred and probably blocked by scarring after such an incision.

PRINCIPLES OF SURGERY FOR TESTICULAR TRAUMA

Blunt trauma to the testes can result in rupture of the tunica albuginea with large hematocele formation and pressure necrosis of the testicle. Early surgical intervention with exploration, drainage, and repair of the injury are indicated.[13, 47] McCormack et al.,[48] in discussing their experience with five cases, emphasize the necessity for early exploration in order to preserve the testicle.

The surgical principles to be followed in treating testicular trauma are (Fig. 11–1): (1) exploration, (2) drainage of the hematocele, (3) excision of any damaged or devitalized tissue, (4) freshening of the edges of the tunica albuginea, (5) closure of the tunica albuginea with absorbable suture mate-

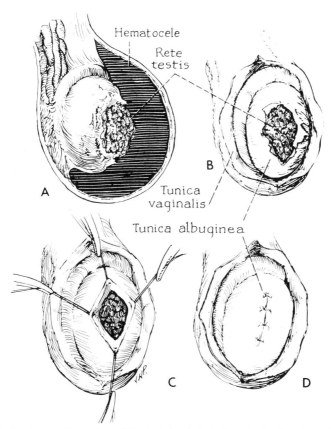

Hematocele

Rete testis

Tunica vaginalis

Tunica albuginea

A

B

C

D

Figure 11-1. Traumatic rupture of the testicle. *A*. Pathology. *B*. Exploration and drainage of hematocele. *C*. Excision of devitalized tissue. *D*. Closure of tunica albuginea. (From McCormack, J. L., Kretz, A. W., and Tocarrtins, R.: J. Urol., 96:80–82, 1966.)

rial after adequate hemostasis has been achieved, and (6) adequate postoperative drainage of the scrotum.

Similar principles should be observed in treating penetrating wounds of the testicle. However, any foreign bodies should be removed if possible.[36] In bullet wounds, scrotal trauma and tissue devitalization will be greater and will require more extensive debridement. Orchiectomy may be necessary if the trauma is so great that preservation of the organ is impossible.

TORSION OF THE TESTIS

Torsion of the testis is a well-known surgical emergency.[1] Early diagnosis is most important, and exploration, relief of the torsion, and bilateral fixation of the testes should be done as soon as possible to preserve testicular viability.

Leape[43] has reported, based on experience with a large series, a maximal safe period of up to 24 hours after the onset of symptoms. We personally feel that one should explore within 6 to 8 hours if spermatogenesis is to be maintained.

Torsion of the testis may occur in undescended testes.[43] An interesting recent report describes a patient with torsion of an intra-abdominal testis with a resultant clinical picture similar to that of acute appendicitis.[21]

We prefer a surgical approach by a high scrotal incision, but inguinal exploration certainly is acceptable. The testicle is explored, and the torsion is relieved by twisting the cord into a normal position. The tunica vaginalis is opened, and moist warm packs are placed on the testicle. If normal color returns to the testicle within 10 to 15 minutes, it is viable. We usually place a running catgut suture around the tunica vaginalis for hemostasis and leave it open.

The testis is then fixed with three separate 0 chromic catgut sutures through the tunica albuginea to the deep scrotal layers. The sutures should be placed in a triangle near one another so that torsion cannot occur again. At the time of exploration the appendix testis is also usually excised to prevent future torsion of that useless appendage.

The procedure must be done bilaterally to prevent future torsion on the contralateral side. Indeed, if an orchiectomy is indicated, because of gangrene secondary to torsion, then fixation of the contralateral testis is mandatory.

CRYPTORCHISM

There is evidence that if a child's testicle remains outside of the scrotum beyond the age of 5 years,[17, 26, 35] irreversible changes begin to take place, and if the testicle remains outside of the scrotum until puberty, it will be incapable of producing sperm thereafter. The intra-abdominal temperature, which is 2° to 3° C. higher than the scrotal temperature, is sufficiently high to prevent normal spermatogenic development (see Chapter 4).

We generally recommend hormone therapy or orchiopexy or both before the child is 5 years old, although there is some evidence that fertility may be preserved even if therapy is started after the age of 9 or 10.[41, 65] Certainly the testis must be in the scrotum before the onset of puberty to allow any chance for future fertility potential.[16]

Hecker and Hienz,[35] in a combined series of 346 patients with unilateral testicular dystopia, noted retained fertility in 120 patients (35 per cent). Gross and Replogle[31] have reported retained fertility at 80 per cent. Some doubts have been raised about the future fertility potential in any case of bilateral cryptorchism. However, we have seen some cases of bilateral orchiopexy prior to puberty in which the patient subsequently demonstrated fertility.

Despite the failure of spermatogenesis to take place in the abdominally located testes, androgenic function and secretion persist owing to continued function of the heat-resistant Leydig cells.

TESTICULAR FIBROSIS

The longer the testes stay within the abdomen, the greater is the testicular fibrosis that occurs. If the testes remain permanently in the abdomen after the age of 30 or 35 not only is spermatogenesis completely absent, but also hormonal secretion is significantly diminished,[42] owing to the fact that total degeneration of the testis may result from complete testicular fibrosis. Fibrosis may be so extensive that a premature failure of androgenic function may be noted as early as 35 to 40 years of age.

NEOPLASIA IN UNDESCENDED TESTES

The incidence of neoplasms in undescended testes is alarmingly high, at least in many reported series. In a series of 510 testicular tumors at Walter Reed Army Hospital, 5.1 per cent were found in cryptorchid testes,[50] and at Memorial Hospital in New York City, 15 per cent of 95 testicular tumors occurred in undescended testes.[20] It is estimated that the frequency of tumors in undescended testes in the young adult is about 45 times as great as that in normally descended gonads. Hormone therapy or orchiopexy should be attempted in order to bring the abdominal testis down to its normal scrotal position. Although the high incidence of malignancy persists, the testis can be easily palpated in the scrotal position, and abnormal growth can be detected more readily.[15, 54]

The fate of the atrophic undescended testis[34] is indeed a problem because of the possibility of malignant degeneration. The presence of two testicles in the scrotum of the prepubertal or pubertal male is probably necessary for proper psychosexual development. This has been emphasized by Gross and Replogle[31] and is another indication for early correction of the undescended testicle.

We feel that a testicle should be in the scrotum. Orchiectomy should be performed if the testicle cannot be placed in its proper position or if it is atrophic or grossly abnormal. Our experience with staged orchiopexy[51] is unfavorable, and we feel that failure of orchiopexy at the time of initial surgery is an indication for orchiectomy.

Undescended testes in adults should be placed in the scrotum or removed. Testicular prostheses may be used if a full scrotum is cosmetically or psychologically desired. The incidence of testicular tumors is low in general (2 per 100,000 men per year), yet an undescended testis produces no sperm and has a high potential to develop malignancy. Certainly the undescended testis should be removed before attempting hormonal stimulation of spermatogenesis in the infertile male with unilateral cryptorchism.

HORMONE THERAPY WITH HCG

Androgens should not be employed at any time in the treatment of cryptorchism. Human chorionic gonadotrophic (HCG) hormone in either a rapid or slow treatment schedule should be used. The rapid method (four injections of 5000 I.U. every second day) has the advantage of producing less development of secondary sexual characteristics. The slow schedule of therapy is given in doses of 500 I.U. three times a week for 3 weeks. If the child is over 10 years old, the dose should be doubled. This method is associated with a greater degree of development of the penis and pubic hair and the occurrence of erections. After therapy the pubic hair may diminish or remain at the same state of development until spontaneous maturation of the testes at the normal time of puberty.

Ehrlich et al.[23] found that descent occurred after hormonal therapy in 23 per cent of 350 patients with undescended testes. The success rate was greater (32 per cent) in patients with bilateral nondescent than in those with unilateral undescended testes (16 per cent). Our own experience with unilateral nondescent is considerably better.

Even if the hormonal therapy does not result in testicular descent, it may make surgical treatment easier because it induces scrotal development and enlarges the cord. These changes facilitate the intravascular dissection that is occasionally necessary to make the cord structures long enough so that the testicle may be placed within the scrotum without tension.

The administration of chorionic gonadotropin also serves another distinct purpose. In the patient with bilateral cryptorchism, it may not be evident whether or not the testes are capable of functioning or whether the gonads are present at all.[2] If the patient with bilateral cryptorchism fails to show any androgenic response to the slow dose regimen described earlier, one may conclude either that no testicular tissue is present at all or that the testicles are so atrophic that they are incapable of function.

Anorchia

Baseline plasma FSH and LH levels should be obtained in patients with anorchia; these will usually be elevated. Following treatment with chorionic gonadotropin, plasma testosterone levels will not rise. These two tests are diagnostic for anorchia. In such a case, if surgical exploration for the testicles is performed, the surgeon is forewarned that the testicles may be absent or undeveloped.

If it is demonstrated that the child does not have functioning testicles, he should have androgen therapy when he reaches puberty to develop his secondary sexual characteristics and to prevent the occurrence of eunuchoidal changes. Such therapy is best left to the endocrinologist.

ASSOCIATED ANOMALIES

An undescended testicle is often associated with other renal or ureteral anomalies, and intravenous pyelography may be indicated if no allergy exists.[46] If renal agenesis is present there is also the possibility of an undescended testis or testicular absence on the ipsilateral side. Bilateral cryptorchism may also be associated with genetic dysplasia such as Klinefelter's syndrome or intersex problems; a buccal smear may be necessary to differentiate these abnormalities.

ORCHIOPEXY

If the testis or testes fail to descend within 2 weeks after the last injection of HCG and some noticeable sexual changes have resulted from the injections, orchiopexy is necessary. This operation should be performed by the urologist. The Bevan technique of orchiopexy is preferred to the two-stage Torek operation because damage to the blood supply of the testicle is likely to occur in the two-stage operation when the testicle is sutured to the subcutaneous tissue of the thigh.

Bevan Technique

The technique of Bevan orchiopexy is as follows.[6, 64] The incision is made above the inguinal ligament from the pubic tubercle toward the flank. Ordinarily an incision of 2 to 4 inches is sufficient. The external oblique muscle is exposed and is incised in the direction of its fibers. The testicle with it fascial layers and tunica vaginalis is then located. If it is not present in the inguinal canal, retroperitoneal or intraperitoneal exploration is indicated. If the testis is intra-abdominal or definitely cannot be brought into the scrotum, orchidectomy should be considered.

The tunica vaginalis is removed from the testis, and gentle retroperitoneal finger dissection is carried out along the cord; the hernia sac which is almost always present is then dissected free and is ligated with silk or chromic sutures. Further dissection is performed in the cord to free its structures and adhesions around the vas deferens, so that proper length of the cord can be achieved to bring the testis into the scrotum. Incision of the transversalis fascia and ligation of the deep epigastric vessels may be necessary to achieve proper cord length.

The scrotum is developed digitally into a thin sac to be ready to receive the testis. A strong silk suture is then brought through the gubernaculum of the testis at its lower pole and is threaded through the bottom of the scrotum, using a straight needle. The silk suture is attached to a rubber band, which is fixed with only slight tension to the thigh of the patient. The external oblique muscle is then closed over the cord with a 2–0 chromic catgut suture, and the skin is closed with interrupted silk or nylon sutures.

We prefer to perform orchiopexy on one side at a time in cases of bilateral cryptorchism. This reduces postoperative morbidity and eliminates the chances of bilateral wound infections that may result in testicular atrophy.

Brendler and Wulfsohn[12] have described an interesting technique in cases of orchiopexy when the cord is too short. This involves temporary clamping of the cord with a rubbershod clamp to determine whether the testis has sufficient collateral circulation to maintain viability. If it does, the cord is transected, leaving the vas and its vessels intact with resultant increase in length.

EPIDIDYMOVASOSTOMY

When the seminal ejaculate is azoospermic but contains fructose, and the testicular biopsy has demonstrated normal spermatogenesis, epididymal obstruction is highly probable. Multiple cystic anomalies of microscopic size and other congenital defects are presently far more common causes of such obstruction than are postinflammatory obstructive lesions resulting from untreated gonorrhea. The fructose test serves to differentiate congenital absence of the ductal system from occlusions of the duct. Complete azoospermia due to tuberculosis is generally not amenable to surgical correction because of the extensive involvement of the epididymides, vasa, and seminal vesicles.

Robert Schoysman of Belgium suggests that there is no necessity for preliminary biopsy of the testis. He feels that the presence of an epididymis distended with sperm as seen under a microscope at the time of exploration is sufficient evidence of active spermatogenesis in the testis and obstruction of the epididymis.[61]

RESULTS

Postinflammatory lesions of the tail of the epididymis offer the best chance for cure. Among patients successfully undergoing this operation, about 20 per cent have been able to achieve pregnancy, and these patients deserve the champagne. Sperm may appear in the ejaculate of a much higher percentage of the patients, however.

Only rare success has been reported in those cases in which azoospermia is due to congenital anomalies rather than to postinflammatory obstruction. Hanley[33] reported only one pregnancy after 83 vasoepididymal anastomoses. In these patients sperm were found in the head of the epididymis, and the vas deferens was patent, but a congenital anomaly of the epididymis was present.

Amelar and Dubin[7] reported 22 cases of azoospermia secondary to epididymal obstruction. Among these 15 patients had a definite history of epididymitis. The other seven patients had congenital epididymal obstruction. Bilateral epididymovasostomy on the 15 patients with epididymitis resulted in eight patients able to produce sperm in their ejaculates, but only four had good semen quality. There were four pregnancies which resulted in three normal children and one early miscarriage. All operations failed in the seven patients with congenital epididymal obstruction.

Getzoff[29] conducted a survey of 150 urologists and published the following tabulation:

Question III EPIDIDYMOVASOSTOMY*

	NO.	PER CENT
I have performed this operation with:		
No success	42	28.0
Rare (1%) success	31	20.7
Occasional (5%) success	32	21.3
Moderate (20%) success	21	14.0
Moderately encouraging success compatible with that reported in the literature (50 to 70%)	4	2.7
Never performed this operation	20	13.3
When the indications are present that lend themselves to an epididymovasostomy:		
I encourage the operation	14	9.3
I discourage the operation	41	27.3
I acquaint the patient with a realistic concept of the procedure and its prognosis	95	63.3

*From Getzoff, P.: Surgical management of male infertility. Results of a survey. Fertil. Steril., 24:553, 1973.

TECHNIQUE

The procedure of vasoepididymal anastomosis was popularized by Hagner[32] and Bayle[11] in 1936. The technique was modified by Humphreys and Hotchkiss in 1939[37] and by Hanley in 1955.[33] The principle of this operation is the anastomosis of a minute elliptical opening in the vas to a similar opening in the epididymis where live sperm have been recovered. The technique that we employ (Fig. 11–2) combines what we believe to be the best features of the Humphreys–Hotchkiss and the Hanley procedures. In this operative procedure the testes epididymides, and spermatic cords

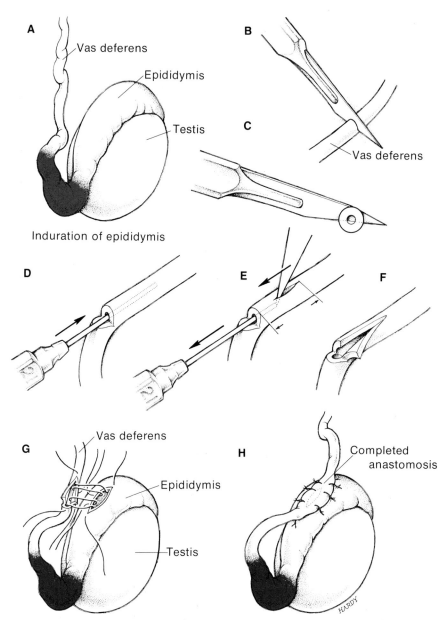

Figure 11–2. Method of epididymovasostomy. *A*. Exposure of anatomy and area of induration and obstruction. *B* to *F*. Method of incision of vas deferens and preparation of the vas for epididymovasostomy. *G*. Vasoepididymal anastomosis using interrupted 6–0 Prolene sutures. *H*. Completed anastomosis.

are exposed through bilateral scrotal incisions. The straight portions of the vasa are identified and are freed from the other cord structures, taking care to avoid devascularization of the vasa. A sufficient length of vas is mobilized so that it can be easily approximated to the epididymis without tension.

Using a number 11 blade, an incision is made into the epididymis at the level of the globus minor on the border opposite its testicular attachment. Any fluid that escapes from the epididymal incision is collected on a sterile glass slide, mixed with a drop of saline, and handed to an assistant outside the sterile field, who places it under the microscope. In favorable cases, many motile sperm will be identified. If sperm are few or absent, another incision is made into the more proximal parts of the epididymis, and the procedure is repeated until a satisfactory site is found for anastomosis.

By making the first exploratory epididymal incision at a point some distance from its most proximal portion, part of the epididymis, as Hotchkiss[37] points out, can be preserved for whatever function it affords the sperm. If the operation fails, a second attempt can be made at a later date, using the remaining proximal areas for a new anastomosis.

Once a favorable site in the epididymis has been selected on each side, the vas is brought adjacent to it, and an incision is made into the vas. An invaluable surgical maneuver for making a clean and adequate incision is to support the vas on the index finger of the left hand while making the transverse incision through the upper portion of the tubular vas with the right hand. The incision should be just deep enough to expose the lumen, and care must be taken not to cut entirely through the vas.

A number 21 hypodermic needle, the tip of which has been honed to blunt its sharp edge, is inserted into the lumen of the distal segment of the vas. A few milliliters of hydrogen peroxide, which has been colored blue with a few drops of indigo carmine, is injected to insure that the vas is patent. The tip of the needle is then withdrawn to a point 0.5 cm. above the transverse incision. The point of the number 11 blade is inserted into the wall of the vas so that it engages the lumen of the blunted end of the needle. Then, as the needle is pulled downward with gentle traction, the knife engaged in the tip of the needle cuts the desired uniform opening through the wall of the vas.

If the blue peroxide solution does not flow easily into the vas, or if there is any doubt about patency, a catheter can be passed into the bladder. If the vas is patent, the urine will be blue. If it is necessary to perform this procedure with the other vas, the bladder will have to be irrigated until the return fluids are clear.

If no solution can be injected into the vas, a silkworm-gut or nylon suture can be passed into the vas as a probe to locate the site of the obstruction. If the obstruction is in an accessible area of the vas, it may be possible to reenter the vas above the point of obstruction and make another test of patency. Occasionally, multiple points of obstruction may be encountered, and if it is not feasible to detour them, the vasoepididymal anastomosis will have to be eliminated on that side.

Anastomosis

Atraumatic number 6–0 Prolene sutures are used for the anastomosis. The sutures are placed through each wall of the incised vas and then deeply into the epididymis in such a manner that all knots are outside the anastomosis. We have found it helpful to use an ocular loupe for better visualization during the placing of these sutures. Some surgeons use an operating microscope during the procedure, but this instrument may be more of a hindrance than a help if the operator is not thoroughly familiar with its use.

At the conclusion of the anastomosis, the scrotal contents are replaced, and the scrotum is closed in two layers with interrupted number 3–0 chromic catgut sutures. Penrose drains are used and are left in place for 24 hours. Sterile dressings and a scrotal suspensory or pressure dressing are applied. The patient may be discharged from the hospital on the fourth or fifth postoperative day.

The procedure of epididymovasostomy is performed on both sides unless the preliminary biopsy has revealed a hopeless condition in one of the testes. On occasion, when the testicle is normal on one side but its vas is occluded, and the opposite testicle is deficient but has a patent vas, a crossed anastomosis has been done successfully. In one such case the patient had unilateral testicular atrophy on the right side and an injured left vas incidental to a difficult low ureterolithotomy, resulting in sterility. At operation, the proximal left vas from the healthy testicle was anastomosed by crossover to the patent distal vas on the right side. He subsequently was found to have good semen quality and has since had two children.

In one case in which the point of obstruction on the right side appeared to be at the ejaculatory duct itself, an attempt was made to release the obstruction by forcible irrigation. All that we succeeded in accomplishing on this side was to blow up the seminal vesicle to enormous proportions, but the blue-tinted radiographic fluid still would not enter the bladder. The temporary seminal vesicle distention was confirmed by radiographic and rectal examinations immediately after the operative procedures. On the left side, however, there was congenital atresia of the epididymis and the convoluted lowermost segment of the vas; the remainder of the vas was patent. A crossed anastomosis was performed in this instance, and sperm were subsequently found in the ejaculum, but so far a pregnancy has not occurred.

When the anastomosis is successful, sperm may be found in the ejaculum within 3 to 6 months; but occasionally it may require up to a year before sperm appear. Periodic follow-up with semen analysis should be performed for at least 1 year before it is determined that the procedure has not been successful.

Splint

The decision of whether or not to use a splint is up to the individual surgeon and will depend on the quality of the anastomosis. Splints are usually left in place for 8 to 10 days. Recently we have eliminated the use of a splint. However, because it may be necessary and useful on occasion, its placement will be described (Fig. 11-3). Once the proper incision has been made into the vas and the needle has been withdrawn, a fine number 0 nylon suture to be used as a splint is passed into the lumen of the distal vas for about 10 cm. The free end of the nylon suture is threaded onto a fine needle, passed through the opening already made in the epididymis, and drawn out about 0.5 cm. distal to the incision. The splint is eventually anchored to the scrotal skin by a button.

It may be found advantageous to use such a splint temporarily as a guide during the accomplishment of the anastomosis, after which it can be removed prior to closure of the scrotum.

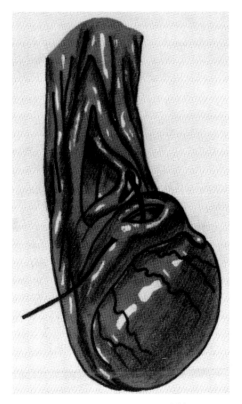

Figure 11-3. Method of splinting in epididymovasostomy.

VASOVASOSTOMY

The restoration of the patency of the vas, in patients who have had a change of heart after previous vas ligation for sterilization, is now being performed more frequently. The probability of success is greater than that in vasoepididymal anastomoses. The chances of restoring functional continuity of the vas are good if the original interruption was not made in the convoluted portion of the vas close to the epididymis. If the obstruction was placed in this convoluted portion, vasovasal anastomosis will be technically difficult, and vasoepididymal anastomosis may be attempted.

Extensive scarring secondary to hematoma or infection at the time of the original vasectomy is also detrimental, and the chances of successful reanastomosis probably vary inversely with the length of vas removed or damaged by electrocoagulation, if that method was used. There is no definite knowledge of the ultimate success of vasovasostomy as related to the time interval between vasectomy and repair; but Schmidt[58] has reported successful reanastomosis as long as 21 years following vasectomy. Phadke and Phadke[53] have also reported success regardless of the length of time between vasectomy and reanastomosis.[53]

Schmidt[59] states that only 0.2 per cent of men undergoing vasectomy seek restoration of fertility. The origin of this figure is somewhat obscure, since adequate data in this area have not been reported. Certainly in our own practice, we have noticed an increasing demand for reversal of vasectomy. The reasons for desiring vas reanastomosis and restored fertility are various: (1) a subsequent marriage (usually to a younger woman) with a desire to have children in this new union; (2) death or severe injury of the patient's children; (3) change of heart in a patient who felt as a young man that sterilization would aid society and "zero population growth"; and (4) psychologic inability to tolerate the concept of being sterile.

RESULTS

In a survey of American urologists,[49] a success rate of 45 per cent was reported for 420 vasovasostomies accomplished by many different splinted and nonsplinted techniques. However, it must be remembered that there is a difference between sperm appearing in the ejaculate and the occurrence of pregnancy.

Hulka and Davis[40] compiled the results from 705 vasovasostomies from the world literature. In 60 per cent of these reappearance of sperm was reported. Lee[45] recently reported 156 cases of vas reanastomosis; 81 per cent of these patients had viable sperm in their ejaculates, but there was a pregnancy rate of only 35 per cent.

Amelar and Dubin performed 93 vasovasostomies, which were followed for at least 1 year. Sperm were present postoperatively in 78 men

(84 per cent). Thirty-one couples had children (a pregnancy rate of 33 per cent).

The reasons for the marked discrepancy between the presence of sperm after vasovasostomy and the pregancy rates remain obscure. Certainly there may be a relationship between fertility and the presence of sperm-agglutinating and immobilizing antibodies in as many as 62 per cent of males tested after vasectomy.[10, 52, 55-57, 63] Significantly high titers (1:32 or greater) of antibodies were found in 18 of 29 men (62.1 per cent) with congenital bilateral absence of the vasa deferentia.[8] Such titers may be related to epididymal obstruction.

High antibody titers *per se* are not a contraindication to surgery, although they may be a poor prognostic sign. We have seen these titers return to normal in some patients following successful vasovasostomy. In others the levels remain elevated.

Semen analyses following vasovasostomy may show sperm as early as 1 month after surgery, but sperm may not appear in some cases until some 6 months later. Poor sperm motility is likely to be noted in the early ejaculates but should be at an adequate level by 6 months. If the semen qualities are poor, further investigation of the patient for other causes of infertility (e.g., varicocele or hormonal imbalance) and appropriate therapy are indicated.

TECHNIQUE

We prefer a technique based on that proposed by Schmidt[59] (Fig. 11–4). The scrotum is well prepared with antiseptic and draped appropriately. The scrotum is then palpated to identify both the scarred area or "granuloma" secondary to the vasectomy and the ends of the vas, if possible. An incision of 2 to 3 inches is then made in the scrotum over this area, and the testis and spermatic cord are delivered from the scrotum. The fascia is incised to expose the scarred ends of the vas, which must be excised. The distal vas is incised, cannulated with a blunt needle, and tested for patency as described earlier in the technique of epididymovasostomy. Spatulation of the distal end may be necessary, since the proximal end is usually dilated and has a greater diameter. The proximal vas is then incised, and fluid from the vas is placed on a microscope slide and examined by an assistant for the presence of sperm. Efforts should be made to prevent spillage of vasal fluid containing sperm into the tissues to prevent granuloma or antibody formation. Vasoepididymal anastomosis should be considered if no sperm are found in the proximal vas.

The two ends of the vas are then grasped with Bonney clamps (Fig. 11–5). A 2–0 nylon suture may be used as a stent while performing the anastomosis but should be removed prior to closure. Eight through and through sutures (we use 6–0 Prolene on a noncutting atraumatic needle) are then

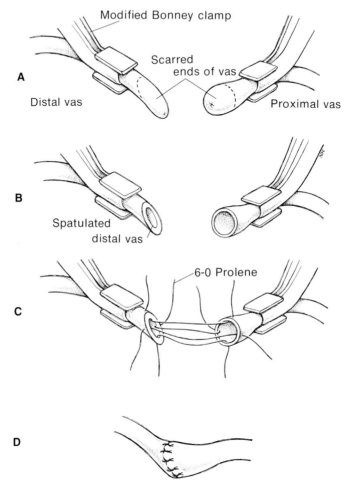

Figure 11–4. Vasovasostomy. *A.* The ends of the vas deferens are exposed and the scarred ends are excised. *B.* After patency has been tested, the distal vas deferens may require spatulation. *C.* Vasovasostomy using interrupted 6–0 Prolene atraumatic sutures. *D.* Completed anastomosis.

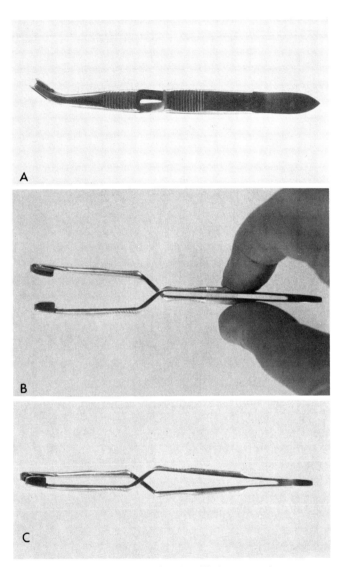

Figure 11–5.   *A*, *B*, and *C*. Modified Bonney clamp.

made with the knots on the outside of the lumen of the vas. The first four sutures are placed at each quadrant, and the remaining four are placed between the quadrant sutures. This gives a closure that aligns mucosa to mucosa and serosa to serosa. The closure is watertight and should not be under tension. Freeing the distal vas will often relieve any possible tension.

The fascia is then closed above the anastomosis. Small indwelling Penrose drains are left, depending on the extent of the surgery, and the skin is closed with catgut sutures. A pressure dressing or scrotal support is then applied.

The operating microscope or ocular magnifying loupe may aid in this meticulous surgery, and familiarity with these instruments is important. Two-layer anastomoses may also be performed, but we have not found this necessary.

EXPERIMENTAL SURGERY

ARTIFICIAL SPERMATOCELE

One of the most frustrating conditions to physicians engaged in the therapy of male infertility is congenital absence of the vasa deferentia. This abnormality accounts for almost 2 per cent of cases of male infertility.[22] It is characterized by normal testes, absent vasa, low semen volume, and absence of seminal fructose and seminal coagulation. Surgical exploration is not necessary to confirm the diagnosis, which can be made with careful physical and seminal examinations.[9]

The testis develops embryologically from the genital ridge on the medial aspect of the mesonephros, while the vas deferens has a different origin from the mesonephric duct. If development is disturbed before the embryo is 13 weeks old, it is possible that a fully developed testis and globus major of the epididymis may occur with an undeveloped vas deferens, seminal vesicle, and ejaculatory duct. If the mesonephric duct ceases to develop at an earlier stage (4 weeks), the ureteric bud does not develop, and the ureter and kidney as well as the vas deferens are absent.[3, 5]

As a practical point, when congenital absence of the kidney is suspected because of nonvisualization on an excretory urogram, an inability to palpate a vas deferens in the scrotum on that side may confirm the diagnosis of renal agenesis.

The treatment of this problem has been frustrating. Testicular biopsy is usually normal, and motile spermatozoa can often be found in the swollen epididymal heads.

Robert Schoysman of Belgium has recently reported his efforts to correct the problem by creation of an artificial spermatocele using a saphenous vein graft.[60, 62] Basically, the operation consists of sewing a saphenous vein graft as a tube to an elliptical incision in the epididymis. In time the graft should distend with epididymal fluid, and the spermatocele can then be aspirated, with the resultant fluid used for artificial insemination of the wife. Epididymal fluid has also been taken at the time of original surgery to be used for direct insemination or preserved by freezing,[38] but no notable success has resulted from these efforts.

Schoysman has reported five pregnancies in 46 patients (10.8 per cent), although 15 patients showed some sperm in the aspirated spermatocele. Using the same technique, Vickers[67] reported two operations in 1975, neither of which led to pregnancy. The main problem is severe fibrosis and scar formation of the graft postoperatively, although sperm-agglutinating antibody problems may also play a role, since they are present in most patients with congenital absence of the vasa.[8]

Amelar and Dubin performed three similar operations using tunica vaginalis as the graft; total fibrosis occurred postoperatively. Charny has recently been using Dacron arterial grafts for the spermatocele but feels that the prognosis is guarded.[18]

INTRAVASAL VALVES

Experimental surgery to preserve fertility after vasectomy by using a valvelike device has been underway under the sponsorship of the Contraceptive Device Branch of the National Institutes of Health. This work is based on the original work of Lee, who was able to create severe oligospermia by occluding the vas, using an intravasal thread.[44] Complete azoospermia and restored fertility were not always achieved with this method. Lee recently stated that he had placed a silicone nylon thread in 544 men.[19] Of 504 patients followed, failures due to vasal dilation or extrusion of the thread were reported in 31. The thread was removed in 42 patients, and sperm reappeared in 35. Silicone plug[39] insertion into the vasa was also attempted with minimal success.

Recent work has been done with rigid and flexible valves. Limited success has been achieved in guinea pigs, rabbits, and dogs, but no successful results have been reported in human beings or primates. One great problem has been the presence of a foreign body in the vas deferens. It has been found that decreased sperm numbers and motility occur when the valves are open even if the valve material is highly nonreactive. Sperm leakage and proper fixation of the device to the vas have also presented problems. The main types of valves under study are: (1) *Freund and Davis,* [28] a rigid gold and stainless steel valve; (2) *Brueschke and Zaneveld,*[14] flexible Silastic valve; (3) *Farcone and Hotchkiss,*[25] dacron plug valve; and (4) *Free,*[27] a molded polymer riod valve.

This brief survey does not cover all the research on valves presently under investigation. We must stress the experimental nature of the work—certainly clinical application does not seem imminent. The repeated

234

surgery necessary for valve insertion and for opening and closing the valves must also be considered should a usable valve eventually be developed.

REFERENCES

1. Aberhart, C.: *In* Campbell, W. (ed.): Urology, 2d ed. Philadelphia, W. B. Saunders Co., 1963, p. 2789.
2. Amelar, R. D.: Anorchism without eunuchism. J. Urol., 76:174, 1956.
3. Amelar, R. D.: Coagulation, liquefaction and viscosity of human semen. J. Urol., 87:187, 1962.
4. Amelar, R. D.: Infertility In Men: Diagnosis and Treatment. Philadelphia, F. A. Davis Co., 1966.
5. Amelar, R. D., and Dubin, L.: Congenital absence of the ductus deferens. J.A.M.A., 213:2080, 1970.
6. Amelar, R. D., and Dubin, L.: Infertility in the male. *In* Practice of Surgery. Vol. 2, Urology. New York, Harper and Row, 1971.
7. Amelar, R. D., and Dubin, L.: Commentary on epididymovasostomy, vasovasostomy and testicular biopsy. *In* Current Operative Urology. New York, Harper and Row, 1975, pp. 1181–1185.
8. Amelar, R. D., Dubin, L., and Schoenfeld, C.: Circulating sperm-agglutinating antibodies in azoospermic men with congenital bilateral absence of the vasa deferentia. Fertil. Steril., 26:228, 1975.
9. Amelar, R. D., and Hotchkiss, R. S.: Congenital aplasia of the epididymides and vasa deferentia: effects on semen. Fertil. Steril., 14:44, 1963.
10. Ansbacher, R.: Vasectomy: sperm antibodies. Fertil. Steril., 24:788, 1973.
11. Bayle, H.: Traitement chirurgical de la stérilité masculine. *In* La Fonction Spermato-genetique du Testicule Humain. Paris, Masson et Cie, 1958, p. 327.
12. Brendler, H., and Wulfsohn, M. A.: Surgical treatment of the high undescended testis. Surg. Gynec. Obstet., 124:605–608, 1967.
13. Brouk, W. S., and Berry, J. L.: Traumatic rupture of the testicle; report of a case and a review of the literature. J. Urol., 52:334, 1944.
14. Brueschke, E. E., and Zaneveld, L. J. D.: Development and evaluation of reversible vas occlusive devices. *In* Sciarra, J. J. *et al.* (eds.): Control of Male Fertility. New York, Harper and Row, 1975, pp. 112–123.
15. Campbell, H. E.: The incidence of malignant growth of the undescended testicle. J. Urol., 81:663, 1959.
16. Charny, C. W.: The spermatogenic potential of the undescended testes before and after treatment. J. Urol., 83:697, 1960.
17. Charny, C. W., and Wolgin, W.: Cryptorchism. New York, Paul B. Hoeber, Inc., 1957.
18. Charny, C. W.: Personal communication.
19. Davis, J. E.: Session summary. *In* Sciarra, J. J. *et al.* (eds.): Control of Male Fertility. New York, Harper and Row, 1975, p. 162.
20. Dean, W. L., and Dean, A. L., Jr.: *In* Campbell, M. F., and Harrison, J. H.: Urology, 3rd ed. W. B. Saunders Co., Philadelphia, 1970.
21. Delinotte, P., Gurly, R., and Hugnet, P.: Case of torsion of an intra-abdominal testis in an adult with bilateral cryptorchidism. J. Urol., 71:97–99, 1965.
22. Dubin, L., and Amelar, R. D.: Etiologic factors in 1294 consecutive cases of male infertility. Fertil. Steril., 22:469, 1971.
23. Ehrlich, B. M., Dougherty, L. J., Tomashefsky, P., and Lattimer, J. K.: Effect of gonado-trophin in cryptorchidism. J. Urol., 102:793–795, 1969.
24. U.S. Department of Defense: Emergency War Surgery. NATO Handbook. Washington, D.C., U.S. Gov. Print. Off., 1958.
25. Farcone, E., Hotchkiss, R. S., and Nuwayser, E. S.: An absorbable intravasal stent and a silicone intravasal reversible plug. Invest. Urol., 13:108–112, 1975.
26. Fonkalsrud, E. W.: Current concepts in the management of the undescended testis. Surg. Clin. N. Amer., 50:847–852, 1970.

27. Free, M. J.: Development of a reversible intravasal occlusive device. *In* Sciarra, J. J. *et al.* (eds.): Control of Male Fertility. New York, Harper and Row, 1975, pp. 124–139.

28. Freund, M., and Davis, J.: New studies with intravasal devices: the gold valve. Presented at the American Urological Association Meeting, St. Louis, Missouri, May 1974.

29. Getzoff, P.: Surgical management of male infertility. Results of a survey. Fertil. Steril., *24*:553, 1973.

30. Gross, M.: Rupture of the testicle; the importance of early surgical treatment. J. Urol., *101*:196, 1969.

31. Gross, R. E., and Replogle, R. L.: Treatment of the undescended testis. Post. Grad. Med., *34*:266–270, 1963.

32. Hagner, F. R.: Operative treatment of sterility in the male. J.A.M.A., *107*:1851, 1936.

33. Hanley, H. G.: The surgery of male subfertility. Ann. R. Coll. Surg., *17*:159, 1955.

34. Hausfeld, K. F., and Schrandt, D.: Malignancy of the testis following atrophy. J. Urol., *94*:69, 1965.

35. Hecker, W. C., and Hienz, H. A.: Cryptorchism and fertility. J. Pediatr. Surg., *2*:513–517, 1967.

36. Hoff, W. G., and Lomax, A. J.: Foreign bodies in the testis. Brit. J. Surg., *55*:255, 1968.

37. Hotchkiss, R. S.: Surgical treatment of infertility in the male. *In* Campbell, M. F., and Harrison, H. H. (eds.): Urology, 3rd ed. Philadelphia, W. B. Saunders Co., 1970, p. 671.

38. Hotchkiss, R. S.: Personal communication.

39. Hrdlicka, J. G., Schwartzman, K. H., and Zinsser, H. H.: New approaches to reversible seminal diversion. Fertil. Steril., *18*:289, 1967.

40. Hulka, J. F., and Davis, J. E.: Vasectomy and reversible vasocclusion. Fertil. Steril., *23*:683, 1972.

41. Karcher, G.: Die Fertilität des behandelten pathologischen Hodenhochstandes unter besonderer Berücksichtigung des Zeitpunktes des hormonellen bzw. operativen Therapie. Langenbecks Arch. Klin. Chir., *317*:288, 1967.

42. Kupperman, H. S.: Human Endocrinology. Philadelphia, F. A. Davis Co., 1963, pp. 504–563.

43. Leape, L. L.: Torsion of the testis: invitation to error. J.A.M.A., *200*:669–672, 1967.

44. Lee, H.: Experimental studies on reversible vas occlusion by intravasal thread. Fertil. Steril., *20*:735, 1969.

45. Lee, H.: Technique and results of vasectomy in Korea. *In* Siarra, J. J. *et al.* (eds.): Control of Male Fertility. New York, Harper and Row, 1975, pp. 76–77.

46. Mayor, D. M.: Commentary on orchiopexy. *In* Whitehead, E. D. (ed.): Current Operative Urology. Philadelphia, Harper and Row, 1975, pp. 1164–1167.

47. McCormack, J. L.: Commentary on traumatic rupture of the testicle. *In* Whitehead, E. D. (ed.): Current Operative Urology. New York, Harper and Row, 1975, p. 1138.

48. McCormack, J. L., Kretz, A. W., and Tocarrtins, R.: Traumatic rupture of the testicle. J. Urol., *96*:80–82, 1966.

49. O'Connor, V. J.: Anastomosis of the vas deferens after purposeful division for sterility. J. Urol., *59*:229, 1948.

50. Patton, J. F., and Mallis, N.: Tumor of testes. J. Urol., *81*:457, 1959.

51. Persky, L., and Albert, D. J.: Staged orchiopexy. Surg. Gynec. Obstet., *132*:43–45, 1971.

52. Phadke, A. M., and Padukone, K.: Presence and significance of auto-antibodies against spermatozoa in the blood of men with obstructed vas deferens. J. Reprod. Fertil., *7*:163, 1964.

53. Phadke, A. M., and Phadke, A. G.: Experience in the reanastomosis of the vas deferens. J. Urol., *97*:888, 1967.

54. Robson, C. J., Bruce, A. W., and Charbonneau, J.: Testicular tumors. J. Urol., *94*:440, 1965.

55. Rümke, P.: Sperm-agglutinating auto-antibodies in relation to male infertility. Proc. R. Soc. Med., *61*:275, 1968.

56. Rümke, P., and Hellinga, G.: Auto-antibodies against spermatozoa in sterile men. Amer. J. Clin. Pathol., *32*:357, 1959.

57. Rümke, P., Van Amstel, N., Messer, E. N., *et al.*: Prognosis of fertility of men with sperm agglutinins in the serum. Fertil. Steril., *25*:393, 1974.

58. Schmidt, S. S.: Anastomosis of the vas deferens: an experimental study. II. Success and failure in experimental anastomosis. J. Urol., *81*:203, 1959.

59. Schmidt, S. S.: Principles of vasovasostomy. Contemp. Surg., *7*:13–17, 1975.

60. Schoysman, R.: La création d'un spermatocele artificiel dans les agenesis du canal deferent. Bull. Soc. R. Belge. Gynecol. Obstet., *38*:307, 1968.
61. Schoysman, R.: Personal communication, 1974.
62. Schoysman, R., and Drouart, J. M.: Progrès récents dans la chirurgie de la stérilité masculine et feminine. Acta Clin. Belg., *71*:261, 1972.
63. Shulman, S., Zappi, E., Ahmed, U., *et al.*: Immunologic consequences of vasectomy. Contraception, *5*:269, 1972.
64. Snyder, W. H., and Greaney, E. M.: Undescended testes. *In* Benson, C. D. *et al.* (eds.): Pediatric Surgery. Vol. 2. Chicago, Year Book Medical Publishers, Inc., 1962, p. 1041.
65. Sohval, A. R.: Histopathology of cryptorchism: a study based upon the comparative histology of retained and scrotal testes from birth to maturity. Amer. J. Med., *16*:345, 1954.
66. Umbey, C. E., Jr.: Experience with genital wounds in Vietnam: a report of 25 cases. J. Urol., *99*:660, 1968.
67. Vickers, M. A.: Creation and use of a scrotal sperm bank in aplasia of the vas deferens. J. Urol., *114*:242, 1975.

Chapter 12

ARTIFICIAL DONOR INSEMINATION (AID)

RICHARD D. AMELAR, M.D.
LAWRENCE DUBIN, M.D.

I. Factors favoring recommendation of AID
II. Choice of couple
III. Choice of donor
IV. Frozen semen
V. Legal aspects of donor insemination

The preceding chapters have emphasized that the diagnosis and treatment of the infertile male must be approached in a rational and orderly manner designed to establish and, when possible, eliminate the causative factors. In spite of all scientific measures, however, there will be couples who are denied a child because the husband's infertility cannot be remedied. When the wife has good fertility potential, donor insemination may often be a happy solution for these couples.*

Artificial insemination with the husband's sperm (AIH) was employed long before artificial donor insemination (AID). John Hunter of England is credited with accomplishing the first insemination of a woman with her husband's semen in 1785. Dr. Marion Sims in this country in 1866 performed 55 inseminations in six women with their husbands' semen. Only one became pregnant. Throughout the 1800s there were reports, especially from Europe, of husband artificial insemination. In the United States, Dr.

---

*A roundtable discussion on artificial donor insemination was held at the home of Dr. Sophia Kleegman in New York City in 1970, shortly before her untimely death.[6] The participants were Dr. Kleegman; Dr. Amelar; Dr. Jerome K. Sherman, a pioneer in developing the technique of freezing human sperm; Dr. Kurt Hirschhorn, a geneticist; and Mrs. Harriet Pilpel, an attorney who is legal counsel for several national organizations whose programs pertain to various aspects of human sexuality. This chapter is based on that roundtable discussion; the material has been reviewed and updated by the participants to include subsequent developments through 1977.

Robert L. Dickenson performed donor insemination in humans with the utmost secrecy, starting in 1890. He was the inspiration and the teacher of all the early practitioners of this therapy and was chiefly responsible for its growing practice and acceptance. Dr. Sophia Kleegman shared his office and practice and became one of the foremost practitioners in the field.

The religious view of the practice has been mixed. The Catholic Church has consistently banned the procedure as adulterous, and the Anglican Church and the Lutheran Church in Sweden also reject donor insemination. Other Protestant denominations have either approved or at least condoned the procedure. No official pronouncement has been made by any branch of the Jewish faith; rabbinic opinions have been cited in individual cases sanctioning donor insemination.[5]

FACTORS FAVORING RECOMMENDATION OF AID

Donor insemination may be recommended in the following situations:

1. When the husband is absolutely sterile (azoospermic or aspermic) or when his semen quality is so poor that he can be considered sterile.

2. When there is severe, intractable oligospermia accompanied by repeated failure with AIH, or when the husband has been unable to obtain a semen specimen for AIH.

3. When the wife is reaching the end of her reproductive years (in her late thirties or early forties) and the husband has such poor semen quality that chances for successful therapy for him are poor. Such couples may want to have a child by AID and then proceed with treatment for the husband; if he improves, the couple can then have a second child fathered by the husband. If his semen quality does not improve with therapy, their second child can be conceived by AID as well.

4. When there is unexplained long-standing infertility in a couple who have a deep desire for parenthood and who have exhausted all other measures.

5. When there is inheritable disease in the husband's line (e.g., Down's syndrome, Huntington's chorea, retinitis pigmentosa, juvenile diabetes, Tay-Sachs disease).

6. When there is Rh incompatibility with a sensitized Rh-negative wife (an Rh-negative donor should be used).

7. When there is intractable infertility with severe sperm auto-agglutination in the husband or persistent wife–husband immunologic incompatibility.

When we encounter a couple in which the husband is absolutely sterile with no hope of improvement, the choice of donor insemination is easy. It is when the husband is not absolutely sterile but has very low fertility potential that the decision to recommend donor insemination is difficult. Generally speaking, we try to do everything medically or surgically possible to improve the husband's semen quality. If the quality cannot be improved to an acceptable level, we try to make optimum use of it by using the better portion of the husband's split ejaculate. A reasonable trial of such procedures should be made but not for more than a year, because the couple may become discouraged and often emotionally distraught if unsuccessful husband inseminations are continued for too long a time.

Other considerations are the age of the wife and the time remaining before her prime childbearing years have passed by. When the husband is almost completely sterile, the doctor can help the couple by advising donor insemination earlier rather than later. Occasionally, the couple may request that the husband's sperm be mixed with that of the donor. This practice should be discouraged because it can reduce the fertility potential of the donor specimen.[9]

In our practice we have encountered three couples who have had a baby of their own after years of infertility and after having a donor baby. In each case the couple were beside themselves with joy. Dr. Kleegman reported seven couples out of almost 500 who had a child of their own after one or two babies from donor inseminations; one couple had two children of their own following a donor baby. In all these families the relationship to the donor baby remained excellent. Interestingly, the poor semen quality of these fathers did not improve; each of them credited his ability to have a child subsequently to the great happiness and relaxation of tensions which the donor baby brought to the marriage.

CHOICE OF COUPLE

It is the physician who is responsible for the choice of both couple and donor. To choose wisely requires more than average ability and experience, and it is essential that the physician have the training to understand human personality and to evaluate the marriage relationship. The ultimate aim of donor insemination is enrichment of the marriage by producing children who are well endowed genetically and are loved, and who will have the opportunity to be assets to the community.

In the choice of couple emotional criteria are of prime importance. Each partner should be well adjusted and feel well married. This is not a means to save a marriage — that is too large a burden to place on any child. An unstable marriage is a definite contraindication to donor insemination. The couple should have a true love of children and should be fully cognizant of the alternative of adoption.

A couple who adopt a baby know relatively little about the mother and even less about the father. Adoption through agencies may be a difficult and drawn-out process, but there are safeguards built into the adoption process intended to protect all concerned. Adoption of babies through private sources may be less difficult and time-consuming, but it also eliminates the safeguards and may be very expensive. Today, because abortion is more freely available, and there is a tendency for unmarried women with babies to keep and rear them, adoptable babies are becoming scarcer. The mother may have been a drug user or may have paid little attention to proper nutritional habits during her unwanted pregnancy. With donor insemination, on the other hand, it is the sperm rather than the baby which has been adopted.

It is most important to investigate the emotional qualifications of the couple. Husband and wife should be interviewed alone, with assurances of inviolable privacy, and then together. The physician must be able to determine how each partner really feels. A husband may explain that he prefers a donor baby because his wife is the woman he chose to be the mother of his children. He too wants to live through the experience of his wife carrying a child, and believes he would feel it to be his own. A conscientious husband who is ambivalent or even secretly opposed may feel that if he cannot give her a baby he has no right to stand in the way of her having her own. Counseling may help him to realize that his first obligation is to the child. Having a child through AID would not add to the couple's happiness and might even hurt the marriage unless the husband has his own need to have children and prefers this solution. Occasionally the husband may confide that he came to the physician against his own desires because he was afraid to oppose his wife. This is a poor environment for a donor baby. Even worse is a domineering wife who has an attitude of hostility and rejection of her husband, in addition to resentment of his infertility.

It is unwise to accept a couple for donor insemination too soon after the husband's infertility has been discovered. He must be given time to recover from the sometimes severe shock of this knowledge. The degree to which each partner can adjust to the situation and to the marriage is a measure of the strength of the bonds between them. This is shown by the statistics collected by Behrman revealing that only 1 of 800 marriages of AID couples ended in divorce.[2]

The medical qualifications of the couple are also important. Dr. Kleegman's usual procedure in selecting a donor was to choose a donor of the same racial and religious group as that of the recipients, with the exception that Christian donors be used for Jewish couples who have had a Tay-Sachs child. Tay-Sachs disease is a genetic disorder which is relentlessly progressive and ultimately fatal. The basic enzymatic defect in this disease, a deficiency of hexosaminidase A, is inherited as an autosomal recessive trait and has a high gene frequency in Ashkenazi Jews. In Ashkenazi Jewish families the incidence of the disease is 1 in 1000 live births, and the gene frequency in these families is 1 in 30. Less well known is the fact that in Sephardic Jews the carrier rate is 1 in 100, and in non-Jews it is 1 in 300. It is therefore mandatory that in the selection of any donor for the couple who have had a Tay-Sachs child, tests must be made to be certain that the donor is not a heterozygote carrier. The heterozygote can be detected by enzymatic assay of serum or skin fibroblasts.[7]

One risk of donor insemination is the possibility that AID children from the same donor (who are therefore half-brothers and half-sisters) might marry and have children, thereby increasing the risk of genetic malformation. However, considering the population and distances involved the chance of such a union is small. It has been estimated that if 2000 children per year were to be born in Great Britain owing to the successful use of AID, and if each donor were responsible for five children, an unwitting incestuous marriage is unlikely to take place more than once in 50 to 100 years.[8] Nevertheless, Beck[1] stresses that, especially when dealing with couples from rural surroundings or small towns, it is incumbent on the physician to make sure that different donors are used, should more than one couple from a given area be seeking help.

Donor insemination has been a source of much happiness. In our urologic practice over the past 20 years we have encountered only one couple in which the husband, after agreeing to donor insemination, had a change of heart shortly afterward and insisted that the wife have an abortion in the second month of her pregnancy, which she did. The couple returned 4 years later more mature and again requested donor insemination. The wife was philosophical about the past, saying that she was glad she had had the experience of achieving a pregnancy and was glad to know she was able to get pregnant. After much reappraisal, the couple looked forward to achieving a second pregnancy.

CHOICE OF DONOR

The results of donor insemination depend not only upon the choice of couple but also on the choice of donor. Both are the physician's responsibility. For appropriate choice of donors, there must be a supply of highly fertile men of superior genetic endowment and intelligence and of varied ethnic and religious backgrounds. Dr. Kleegman preferred to use as donors healthy married medical students or physicians whose wives had healthy children. She refused the request of the occasional couple who preferred to use a friend or relative as the donor since there was too great a risk of serious emotional problems subsequently.

FROZEN SEMEN

The use of frozen semen is one of the great advances in making artificial donor insemination more widely available. Two hundred years ago, Spallanzini was perhaps the first to report observations on the effects of freezing temperatures on human spermatozoa, and Montegazza in 1866 was the first to suggest banks for frozen human semen. During the period 1938 to 1945, it was observed that some human spermatozoa could survive freezing and storage at temperatures as low as minus 269° C. The possibility of preserving sperm by freezing for prolonged periods subsequently arose from the successful use of glycerol as a cryoprotective agent with mammalian spermatozoa in 1949.

However, cryopreservation was largely used for the semen of farm animals, and research on developing techniques applicable to human semen was consequently neglected. It was not until 1953 and 1954 that Sherman and his co-workers reported successful research with human semen, along with the first demonstration that frozen human spermatozoa were capable of fertilization that led to subsequent normal embryonic development. About 25 births resulting from frozen human semen were reported in the next 9 years. From 1953 to 1964, following evaluation of various cryobiological factors, Sherman developed a simple, practical method of preserving human spermatozoa employing liquid nitrogen at a temperature of minus 196° C. Semen pretreated with 10 per cent glycerol by volume was frozen in glass ampules, suspended in the vapor of liquid nitrogen, and subsequently stored in the same container. An average survival of 70 per cent, based upon the number of moving cells, was realized. No further loss was noted during frozen storage for periods of up to a year, after which the semen was thawed in a room temperature water bath. Initial clinical application of this method led to four normal births.

Essentially the same method is used in the semen banks now in operation. Modifications in procedure (for example, use of different diluents or protective substances and electronically controlled cooling) have been introduced by some workers in progressive steps; these may eventually lead to further reduction in loss of motile sperm cells induced by frozen storage. Approximately 1000 births have resulted so far from semen preserved by freezing.[10] However, it has been the experience of clinicians that the fertility capacity of frozen human semen is not as good as that of fresh semen. The frequency of pregnancies that may be expected after inseminations with frozen semen is approximately two-thirds of that expected from fresh semen.[1, 3, 4]

Frozen sperm can now be readily transported great distances in containers of portable liquid nitrogen, making donor insemination more widely available.

The prediction of rapid growth for commercial frozen semen banks has not been realized. To the contrary, there have been cancellations of planned openings of new branches and closing of some existing branches. The explanation given by some commercial banks is that the expected acceleration of activity in prevasectomy storage of semen has never materialized.

The disappointing rate of development in semen banking is due to more than a simple miscalculation. The chief reason appears to be the reluctance of the layman and the medical community to accept the safety of frozen stored human spermatozoa; public statements in 1972 by a task force committee of the American Public Health Association and Planned Parenthood–World Population raised the awesome possibility of genetic damage and birth defects after prolonged frozen storage of human semen. Dr. Kurt Hirschhorn, a geneticist, feels that this possibility will not be resolved until scientists have had the opportunity to study a few thousand successful pregnancies.[6]

LEGAL ASPECTS OF DONOR INSEMINATION

Many legal questions arise in connection with the act of artificial insemination by donor sperm.* In the first place many legal problems affect the child who is the result of artificial insemination. Is the child legitimate in the legal sense? Does the husband have an obligation to support the child? What are the rights of the child in relation to both the husband and the donor in regard to such matters as inheritance?

Unfortunately, there are no real answers to any of these questions. In researching the very small body of law that is involved, it is apparent that questions of legitimacy and support obligations have been decided both ways, and the question of inheritance rights depends in large part on how the question of legitimacy is answered. In other words, if the child is not legitimate the chances are that it has either no inheritance rights or fewer inheritance rights than a legitimate child. However, the United States Supreme Court has decided in *Levy vs. Louisiana,* 1968 that it is not constitutionally permissible to penalize either illegitimate children or their mothers in regard to benefits given by the state. This case may not only affect the inheritance rights of illegitimate children, but also clarify the rights of AID children as well.

In addition to the legal status of the child, donor insemination raises questions of legal importance to the husband. If the husband does not consent to or does not have knowledge of the artificial insemination of his wife by a donor, there are legal arguments in some cases to the effect that the wife has been adulterous and that the husband can sue her for divorce on those grounds. If there is proof of the husband's consent, the chances are that he would be held not to have any right to object or to disclaim the child as his own.

Another legal basis for defeating any disavowal of the child by a husband derives from the presumption of legitimacy. Arguably, when a husband consents to donor insemination, he is precluded from questioning the legitimacy of the child; moreover, he could be held *de facto* to have

---

*This material has been brought up to date by Mrs. Pilpel and her colleague Mrs. Eva Paul.

adopted the child if after the child was born he treated it as if it were his own.

The wife is in some legal jeopardy if the insemination was done without her husband's knowledge and consent. However, faced with an absence of guidelines and precedents, some courts have decided that in some instances the wife was guilty of adultery even though her husband consented.

The legal waters are even more murky in regard to the rights and obligations of the donor. He should not know the recipient of his semen, nor should the husband and wife know who the donor is. Practically speaking, therefore, the risk of the donor incurring either obligation or punishment should be minimal. If the husband, wife, and donor do know each other's identities, legal complications may result. For example, if the child conceived by artificial insemination becomes very wealthy, and if the donor has been selling his sperm because, although healthy and virile, he is impecunious, he might want to claim the right to inherit from the child as if he were the child's parent. An AID child might wish to make a similar claim with respect to the donor. Theoretically, the donor also could be charged with adultery, although this is not known to have happened.

Doctors who perform donor inseminations have been extremely courageous and ethically responsible, according to Mrs. Pilpel. One of the main problems is what should he put on the birth certificate if the doctor knows that the child is the result of artificial insemination. If the donor's sperm has been mixed with the sperm of the husband it would be difficult to state categorically that the doctor had falsified the records by naming the husband as the father of the child. Several years ago a physician in England was jailed for 3 years for falsifying records in a case of artificial insemination by donor sperm. The name of the husband on the birth certificate was considered a falsification.

The American Medical Association has stated that in its opinion no act is illegal unless prohibited by a specific law, written or unwritten. Certainly there is no law against artificial insemination. With reference to donor insemination the director of the Legal Division of the AMA further explains, "I personally doubt very seriously that we have the authority in the American Medical Association to say to the physicians of America that you can or cannot properly engage in this practice. The rights of many people are involved. Meanwhile, until there is legislation, the physician who performs the insemination, the husband, the wife, the child, and the donor are all in an unsatisfactory position with respect to the law."[6] Fortunately, there is a difference between an "illegal" position and an "unsatisfactory" one. On balance, the relevant authorities do not appear to indicate that this is an illegal procedure at present.

The Department of Health of the City of New York adopted a provision in its Sanitary Code in 1947[11] which requires prospective donors of semen to undergo a thorough physical examination. Tests for venereal infection must be made, and freedom from hereditary diseases must be ascertained. The Rh factor of the patient and the donor must be identical. Physicians performing artificial insemination are required to fill out a form indicating the particulars of the insemination. This information is confidential and is available only on authorization of the Health Department.

Subsequently, at least nine states have enacted specific legislation on the subject of artificial insemination. Statutes in New York,[12] Kansas,[13] North Carolina,[14] Oklahoma,[15] Georgia,[16] and Connecticut[17] provide that any child born to a married woman by means of artificial insemination with her consent and that of her husband will be considered the legitimate natural child of the husband and wife for all legal purposes. In Arkansas,[18] a statute provides that a child born following artificial insemination of a married woman with the consent of her husband will be treated as their own child for purposes of intestate succession (i.e., in cases where a valid will does not exist). A California statute[19] provides that the husband of a woman who bears a child as a result of artificial insemination to which he consented is responsible for all necessary food, clothing, shelter, and medical attendance for that child. This statute codifies the result of a decision of the California Supreme Court in the leading case of *People vs. Sorenson*.[20] Maryland has adopted a statute[21] providing that no person shall be required to perform or participate in any artificial insemination procedure. Some of these state statutes require that artificial insemination be performed only by a licensed physician, but none contain the medical safeguards of the New York City Sanitary Code.

The statutes of Georgia, Kansas, New York, North Carolina, Oklahoma, and Connecticut have the important effect of establishing beyond dispute the legitimacy of the offspring resulting from artificial insemination.

When doctors undertake artificial insemination by donor, they should have carefully drawn documents signed by the donor, the husband, and the mother, which make clear not only that each of them understands the process and consents to it but also that the doctor has made no representation which subsequently he can be charged with not carrying out. Particularly in the light of prospects for genetic planning, it would be unfortunate if a doctor said that a child would turn out to be a latter-day Mozart and instead he turned out to be tone deaf.

The office of the General Counsel of the American Medical Association points out that, as in other medical procedures, the physician cannot free himself from the obligation to use due care and skill in the performance of artificial donor insemination. Medicolegal consent forms published by the AMA[22] are suggested for the protection of the physician performing artificial donor insemination.

Although the possibility of a suit by the donor's wife is remote, her written consent to the donation of the semen may also be desirable inasmuch as her marital interests are affected.

Dr. Kleegman in private practice performed artificial donor insemina-

---

Form Q-1

CONSENT TO ARTIFICIAL INSEMINATION

A.M.
Date_____ Time_____P.M.

We, _____ and _____, being hus-
band and wife and both of legal age, authorize Dr._____
and such assistants as he may designate, to inseminate the wife
artificially, and to use the semen of (the husband) (the husband
and a donor or donors) (a donor or donors) for this purpose. We
authorize him to employ such assistants he may desire to assist
him.

We understand that even though the insemination may be repeated as often as recommended by Dr._____,
there is no guarantee on his part or assurance that pregnancy or
full term pregnancy will result.

We agree to rely upon the sole discretion of Dr._____
in the selection of qualified donors and never to seek to discover
the identity of any donor. We agree that following the insemination,

Dr. _____ may destroy all records and information
concerning the identity of the donor or donors.

We, and each of us, acknowledge our obligation to care for and
support and otherwise treat any child born as the result of such
artificial insemination in all respects as though it were our natural
born child.

We understand that if pregnancy shall result, there is the possibility of complications of childbirth or delivery, or the birth of an
abnormal infant or infants, or undesirable hereditary tendencies of
such issue, or other adverse consequences.

(CROSS OUT ANY WORDS ABOVE WHICH DO NOT APPLY)

Signed_____
(Husband)

Signed_____
(Wife)

Witness_____

Figure 12–1. Reprinted from Medicolegal Forms with Legal Analysis, copyright 1973 by the American Medical Association.

Form Q-3

OFFER TO SERVE AS A DONOR OF SEMEN

A.M.
Date_____ Time_____P.M.

To Dr. _____:

1. I offer my services as a donor of semen with the understanding that the identity of any recipient shall not be disclosed to me, nor shall you voluntarily reveal my identity to any recipient.
2. To the best of my knowledge:
   (a) I am in good health; I have no communicable disease; and I do not now, nor have I ever suffered, from any physical or mental impairment or disability, whether inherited or as a result of any disease or ailment, except as follows:

   _____.

   (b) I am not now nor have I ever been afflicted with syphilis

   or any other venereal disease, except as follows:_____

   _____.

   (c) None of my grandparents, parents, brothers, sisters, or children, if any, nor their lineal descendants, have ever been afflicted with emotional illness or any inherited mental or physical disabilities or disease, except as fol-

   lows:_____.

3. For the purpose of determining whether I am acceptable as a donor of semen, I consent to a physical examination, including the taking of blood and other body fluids, by you or any other physician whom you may designate.

Signed_____
(Donor)

Witness_____

Figure 12-2. Reprinted from Medicolegal Forms with Legal Analysis, copyright 1973 by the American Medical Association.

Form Q-5

CONSENT OF WIFE OF DONOR

Date_____

To Dr. _____:

1. I have read my husband's offer to serve as a donor of semen and to the best of my knowledge the statements he has made are true.

2. If my husband is accepted as a donor, I understand that it is your intention to use his semen for purposes of artificial insemination, but not with respect to myself.

3. I know that artificial insemination is a medical procedure intended to cause pregnancy through the use of semen introduced by means other than sexual intercourse.

4. I agree that I shall not attempt to discover the identity of any recipient of my husband's semen.

5. In serving as a donor of semen, I know that my husband may become the father of a child or children of which I am not the mother, but I nevertheless consent to the performance of such services by him.

Signed_____

Witness_____

Figure 12–3. Reprinted from Medicolegal Forms with Legal Analysis, copyright 1973 by the American Medical Association.

tion for about 700 couples, of whom almost 500 had babies (there were three sets of twins). She had the couple sign a consent sheet of which she kept the only copy. This was kept in a safety vault and was thus preserved as legal protection for the child, the couple, and the physician. (Incidentally, when Dr. Kleegman died, her records passed on to the trust of her physician partner.) She felt that the record's main value was to insure that should there be a later marital conflict leading to legal action, neither the husband nor wife could claim that donor insemination was done without the knowledge and consent of both. The couple was advised not to share their plans with any friend or relative and to keep no memo among their papers about the treatment. She felt that legal adoption was ill-advised, a view shared by other practitioners. Dr. Kleegman had no legal problems between the couples and herself as physician. She cited one case in which there was a divorce when the child was 4 years old, but the husband remained a devoted and generous father to the child and is now a grandfather. The mother was wise enough to support this good relationship even when 18 years after the divorce, she remarried and had a child with her new husband.

As to the birth certificate, Dr. Kleegman stated that physicians who inseminate the woman and then deliver her should not hesitate to record the husband as the child's father, and secrecy concerning the insemination should be carefully preserved. Many of her patients came from a distance, and they were advised not to disclose to their local obstetrician how the pregnancy was achieved since it had no bearing on the obstetric care.

Physicians who undertake this therapy feel that their precautions in this regard are ethically justified since their purpose is the protection of the well-being of the child and the family.[1]

Donor insemination helps the wife of the sterile or infertile man to achieve emotional and biological fulfilment as a mother. We have also observed that the husband often welcomes the procedure as an ego-saving device that is preferable to adoption, in which he would have to declare himself unable to procreate. Based on Dr. Kleegman's 40 years of experience, including excellent follow-up over a period of years for many of her babies, artificial donor insemination is a therapeutic measure which can be entirely beneficial if carried out within the framework presented in this chapter. Because each child is a wanted child the families and therefore the community are enriched.

REFERENCES

1. Beck, W. W., Jr.: A critical look at the legal, ethical and technical aspects of artificial insemination. Fertil. Steril., *27*:1, 1976.
2. Behrman, S. J.: Artificial insemination. *In* Behrman, S. J., and Kistner, R. W. (eds.): Progress in Infertility, 2d ed. Boston, Little, Brown & Company, 1975, p. 779.
3. Behrman, S. J., and Sawada, Y.: Heterologous and homologous inseminations with human semen frozen and stored in liquid nitrogen refrigeration. Fertil. Steril., *17*:457, 1966.
4. Chong, A. P., and Taymor, M. L.: Sixteen years' experience with therapeutic donor insemination. Fertil. Steril., *26*:791, 1975.
5. Gordon, J. A., Amelar, R. D., Dubin, L., and Tendler, M. D.: Infertility practice and orthodox Jewish law. Fertil. Steril., *26*:480, 1975.
6. Kleegman, S. J., Amelar, R. D., Sherman, J. K., Hrischhorn, K., and Pilpel, H.: Artificial donor insemination. A round table discussion. Medical Aspects of Human Sexuality, *4*:85, 1970.
7. McKhann, G. M.: GM$_2$ gangliosidosis with hexosaminidase A deficiency. *In* Bergsma, D. (ed.): Birth Defects Original Article Series, Atlas and Compendium. Baltimore, The Williams and Wilkins Company, 1973, pp. 449–450.
8. McLauren, A.: Biological aspects of A.I.D.. (Ciba Foundation Symposium 17) Amsterdam, Elsevier Publishing Company, 1973, p. 3.
9. Quinlivan, W. L. G., and Sullivan, H.: Effect on donor semen of husband's seminal plasma during artificial insemination. Presented at annual meeting of American Fertility Society, Las Vegas, Nevada, April 8, 1976.
10. Sherman, J. K.: Clinical use of frozen human semen. Transplant. Proc. *8*(2) Suppl. 1, 165–170, 1976.
11. New York City Sanitary Code, Section 112, Article 21, Sections 01,03,05 and 07, 1947.
12. New York Domestic Relations Law, Section 73.
13. Kansas Statutes, Sections 23–128, 23–129, and 23–130.
14. North Carolina General Statutes, Section 49 A–1.
15. Oklahoma Statutes, Title X, Sections 551, 552, 553.
16. Georgia Code, Section 74–101.1.
17. Connecticut Public Act No. 75–233.
18. Arkansas Statutes, 61–141.
19. California Penal Code, Title 1X, Section 270.
20. Cal. Rptr. 7 (1968).
21. Maryland Code, Article 43, Section 55E.
22. Medicolegal Forms with Legal Analysis. Chicago, Office of the General Counsel, American Medical Association, 1973.

INDEX

Note: Page numbers in *italics* indicate illustrations; t indicates tables.

251

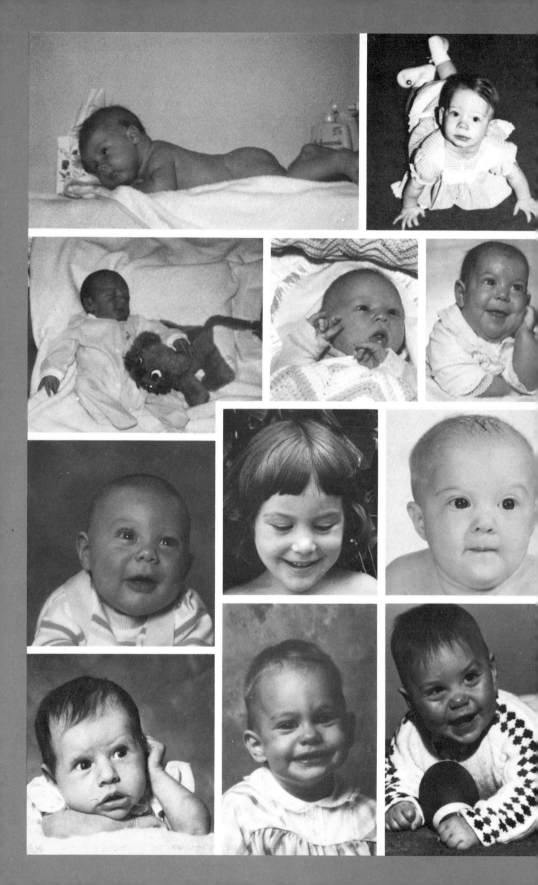